BOOZE TO BALANCE

A LIVER-CENTERED PLAN FOR HEALTH AND HAPPINESS BEYOND DRY JANUARY

THE 30- DAY LIVER HEALING DETOX CHALLENGE

DR. KIM MAKOI

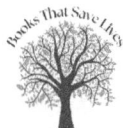

Books That Save Lives

CONTENTS

Foreword   vii

Introduction   ix

A Note from the Author   1

1. Day 1: It Begins   3
2. Day 2: Going with the Flow   6
3. Day 3: Secrets of Motion   10
4. Day 4: The Liver Bank   14
5. Day 5: Liver Emotions?   20
6. Day 6: Gratitude   24
7. Day 7: Slow It Down   27
8. Day 8: Only the Best   30
9. Day 9: Less is More   33
10. Day 10: Mindfulness   36
11. Day 11: Under Pressure   40
12. Day 12: Can't Versus Don't   44
13. Day 13: Breath of Life   47
14. Day 14: Breath of Life (Part 2)   51
15. Day 15: Liver Posture?   54
16. Day 16: Positive Liver Emotions   58
17. Day 17: FAST   61
    Bonus Balance   65
    Homeopathy
18. Day 18: Fire it Up!   67
19. Day 19: Cool it down   70
    Bonus Thoughts   73
    Kitchen Gear
20. Day 20: Fletcherize it!   75
    Bonus Thoughts   79
21. Day 21: Stop the Presses!   81
22. Day 22: Beet It!   83

Bonus Recipe   86
Green Smoothie

23. Day 23: The Dark Crystal   88
Bonus Thoughts   91
24. Day 24: The Bitter Truth   93
25. Day 25: Backyard Bounty   96
Bonus Thoughts   101
26. Day 26: Allergens   103
27. Day 27: Oil it Up   106
28. Day 28: Skin Deep   110
Bonus Thoughts   113
Liver Spots

29. Day 29: The Sugar Thing   115
Shameless Self-Promotion   119
About That Sugar Thing...

30. Day 30: Graduation Day   121
31. Bonus Chapter: The (In)Famous Liver Flush   124

About Books That Save Lives   135

FOREWORD

When I first encountered Booze to Balance, I felt like I was reading the work of a kindred spirit—someone who understands that true healing doesn't happen through restriction and shame, but through empowerment, education, and love for the body we live in.

Dr. Kim Makoi has taken one of the most misunderstood organs in the human body—the liver—and lovingly handed it the microphone. And what a voice! This book is practical, compassionate, and refreshingly funny. It doesn't lecture—it liberates.

As a chronic disease reversal specialist and advocate for root-cause healing, I've spent years teaching people that food is medicine, that chronic illness is often reversible, and that the human body is wired for regeneration and restoration when given the right conditions. What Dr. Kim has done here is take that same philosophy and apply it through a lens that's often neglected: our relationship with alcohol, sugar, and the emotional weight that can build up in the tissues when we're out of balance.

This isn't just a "liver detox." It's a wake-up call wrapped in humor and kindness. You'll learn how to hydrate better, breathe deeper, chew slower (hello, Fletcherizing!), and rethink the way you relate to comfort foods and coping mechanisms. And most importantly, you'll feel seen—no guilt trips, just guidance.

Dr. Kim has a rare gift for making complex wellness concepts approachable—and even joyful. His 30-day challenge format invites you in without overwhelm, making change feel not only possible but exciting. The stories, the analogies (trust me, you'll never look at a Zapper or a dandelion the same way), and the heartfelt encouragement make this one of the most human health books I've read in a long time.

If you're ready to reset your relationship with your liver, your habits, and your health—this book is your new best friend. You're in excellent hands.

Let the healing begin.

With gratitude and green juice,

Dr. Nicolette Richer, DSocSci
Founder & CEO, Richer Health Consulting Ltd. & Green Moustache Organic Cafes

Author of Eat Real to Heal: Using Nutrient Dense Foods for Longevity and Happiness

INTRODUCTION

Some books are born on bestseller lists. Others sneak out the back door under a fake name, hoping no one notices.

This book was the latter.

Originally created as a quirky little gift for the handful of folks who took my online course during the Zoom boom of 2022, Booze to Balance was never intended for the spotlight. It started as a course for my chiropractic patients—many of whom came in for stubborn neck and shoulder pain that just wouldn't budge. When the usual treatments didn't help, I dug deeper and noticed a pattern: a low-grade stress on the liver and blood sugar systems that was quietly undermining their healing.

These weren't folks with dramatic diagnoses or alarming lab results. But they were stuck. In pain. Tired. Sluggish. Foggy. A little more inflamed than they should be. And sometimes... craving just one more drink to take the edge off.

People are so tired of throwing pills at problems – even if those pills are "just" nutritional supplements! So, I created a pill-free program to help them reset. To my surprise (and delight), people weren't just feeling better physically— they were drinking less alcohol without even trying. The feedback was consistent:

"I'm drinking way less... and I wasn't even trying!"

"I've been trying to cut down for years, and nothing really worked until this

"Why does no one talk about liver health when we talk about drinking?"

Exactly.

This is not an anti-alcohol manifesto. It's not about shame, blame, or giving up every pleasure in life. It's about tuning in to your body and supporting your system—especially your poor, overworked liver—so you don't need the nightly glass (or three) just to feel okay.

It's about feeling good in your body again.

And this time, I'm putting my real name on it.

Because even though it started as a little side project for "my" people, I now realize this message deserves a wider reach. And as fate would have it, after a serendipitous meeting at the San Francisco Writers Conference, I found a publisher who believed the same thing, too! (Thanks, Brenda!)

Booze to Balance is for anyone who's tried the usual approaches and felt like something was missing. It's for people who want to feel better without being lectured. It's for people who are ready for real change—but on their own terms.

So, whether you're here to cut back, clean up, or just get curious—welcome. I hope this book helps you feel more balanced, less inflamed, and more at home in your body.

Cheers (yes, cheers) to that!

— Dr. Kim

A NOTE FROM THE AUTHOR

TO GET the most out of this book, I recommend taking it one day at a time. It's arranged as a 30-day challenge, with daily steps designed to guide you toward your goals. While you *could* read it straight through, I think you'll have the best experience if you treat it like a journey, not a race!

Now, before we dive in, I should probably clear something up right away so nobody gets their panties in a twist: I'm not a medical doctor, and this is *not* medical advice! If you have a medical condition, please consult your medical doctor or licensed healthcare provider. The information in this book is purely informational and intended for basic wellness purposes, not to diagnose or treat any specific medical issues. Don't hurt yourself, okay?

So, if we're just talking about general wellness—and not "treating a medical condition"—you might be wondering, "Why the liver? That sounds pretty specific, doesn't it?"

Well, yeah, it is specific, but for good reason! The liver comes up *all the time* in my practice—and not just in mine, but in healthcare across the board. Non-alcoholic fatty liver disease, for example, is rampant these days. When I was growing up, it was pretty rare. But modern life is tough on the liver—from the food we eat to the products we use, and even to our sedentary lifestyles.

And let's not forget the emotions traditionally associated with the liver and gallbladder: anger, resentment, frustration, depression, indecision... Sound familiar?

Let's face it, we live in some seriously "livery" times!

That's why we're starting here.

DAY 1: IT BEGINS

TODAY'S THE DAY! We're kicking off the 30-day Liver Challenge!

Chances are, if you're on this journey, it's not your first health rodeo. You've probably been thinking about your liver for a while now—and tried a few things to give it a boost. Sure, diet makes a difference (including cutting back on the booze) but the real challenge is staying healthy while still living your life in the real world, right?

Over the next 30 days, you'll pick up skills and tools to support your liver health—without having to hit "pause" on your life.

But first, let's talk goals and accountability.

People with goals get better results. And when those goals are written down? Even better! Add accountability, and you've got a recipe for success.

A good goal is specific, measurable, and attainable. For liver health, it could be anything from improving a lab result to dropping a few inches around your waist. It might even be better sleep!

Many people with liver stress also feel tightness or tenderness under their ribs on the right side. If that's you, try this: take a deep breath in, then blow it all out, and as you're blowing out, gently press the fingertips of both hands underneath the edge of your ribcage on one side. Do this for a few breaths, pay attention to what it feels like, and then repeat the process on the other side.

Did you notice a difference between the two sides? Did one side feel like squishy pressure, while the other side felt tight, tender, or just more "sensitive?" That squishy pressure is totally normal—your organs are soft, and it should feel like relaxed pressure when you press in on them. You shouldn't feel any pain, though. If the right side feels tighter or more sensitive, that could be a sign your liver is under some stress. In that case, a great goal for this challenge would be to balance out that tightness or sensitivity over the next 30 days.

Next: accountability.

Each day, you'll get a simple step to complete. To stay on track, it's important to have an accountability consequence—what happens if you don't complete the day's step? Studies show that negative consequences work better than positive ones. For example, promising to donate to a cause you *dislike* might motivate you more than rewarding yourself with a treat! Find a consequence that really stings, and you'll be more likely to stick to your plan.

Today's assignment has 2 parts. The first is to come up with your GOAL for this challenge. The second is to decide on what your ACCOUNTABILITY consequence will be if you do not follow through.

What is it that your toxic or stressed-out liver is preventing you from doing or being? What do you want to achieve and why? Set a timer for 25 minutes and decide on a clear and measurable goal for your liver loving challenge. Next, set an accountability consequence for if you fail to take the action steps to get to the goal.

BJ Palmer, the developer of chiropractic, once said, "Is life worth living? That depends on the liver!" Give your liver a little pat (it's located behind the lower front ribs on the right side of your torso) and get ready to live better!

P.S. You can always DM me on LinkedIn and let me know what your goals and accountability consequences are!

DAY 2: GOING WITH THE FLOW

WE OFTEN THINK of the liver as a waste station, or something dirty that needs to be cleaned out. But that's not the case. The liver is an incredible organ with countless functions that help keep the body running smoothly!

Let's start with one simple structural fact about the liver: it's full of little tubes! These include veins, arteries, and biliary ducts. The veins deliver low-oxygen blood back to the heart, the arteries bring fresh, oxygen-rich blood to the liver, and the biliary ducts carry bile from the liver to the gallbladder.

The health of these tubes is crucial to liver function!

Now, if you've got tubes that deliver fluids, what's one thing you know can make or break their health? The thickness of the fluid.

Thicker fluids can lead to slow flow, clogs, and blockages.

So, what's one obvious way to reduce the thickness of a fluid? By diluting it!

When you're well-hydrated, your blood is less thick and less prone to clots. Staying hydrated has even been shown to reduce the risk of stroke and help in stroke recovery. Improving blood flow to and through the liver makes a huge difference in how well your liver functions.

The same goes for bile. When you're hydrated, bile can flow easily. But if bile becomes too thick, it can clump in the gall-bladder and lead to gallstones. Yikes!

So, hydration is key.

You probably know the basic rule of thumb for water intake: about 1 quart for every 50 pounds of body weight per day, or 1 liter for every 23 kg. For most adults, this means drinking 2-3 quarts or liters of water each day.

That's a lot of water! And while some people have no problem drinking that much, others might struggle. Ever feel like you're just peeing it out as fast as you drink it? If that's you, it means your body isn't absorbing the water properly.

The most common cause? Electrolyte imbalance.

To help solve this, try adding a pinch of raw, unrefined salt (like Celtic sea salt or pink Himalayan salt) to your water. This can help your body absorb the water better, and you might not need to drink as much. Don't worry—raw salt contains trace minerals that won't negatively affect your blood pressure the way processed white table salt does. (note: always consult your medical doctor if you're taking blood pressure medication!)

Boost hydration with gel-forming foods.

Another way to improve hydration is by incorporating gel-forming foods into your diet. These foods store water and slow absorption, making hydration more effective. Ground chia seeds are especially great for this—add them to your morning smoothie to significantly boost hydration.

Desert-dwelling cultures around the world often start their day with a smoothie to make the most of the limited water they have available. You can do the same to supercharge your hydration!

Other gel-forming foods include apples, which contain soluble fiber called pectin. For liver health, go for a green apple, as the sourness is especially beneficial for supporting the liver and gallbladder.

A healthy liver needs proper hydration.

Which hydration strategy will you commit to for the next 30 days?

- Will you drink 2-3 quarts or liters of water per day, based on your body weight? (Tip: Try to drink your first quart before noon to prevent an afternoon energy crash!)
- Will you add raw salt to your water 2-3 times a day?
- Will you start each day with a smoothie that includes ground chia seeds?
- Will you add more soluble fiber to your diet, like green apples?

Make it specific and measurable so you can stay committed!

Today's Assignment: Choose one (or more) hydration strategies to focus on for the next 30 days.

If hydrating is new to you, you may want to track your water intake in a journal or phone app to make sure you're staying on target. And don't forget—if you drink anything dehydrating (like alcohol or coffee), add an extra glass of water to balance it out!

3

DAY 3: SECRETS OF MOTION

WELCOME TO DAY 3!

Yesterday, we focused on making sure the blood and bile flowing through your liver can move optimally. Hydration is a big part of that—whether it's from drinking water or eating hydrating foods. But today, we're going to explore a part of your body's hydration system you might not have heard much about: the fascia!

What's fascia?

Fascia is a thin, continuous sheet of tissue that covers every organ, muscle, bone, blood vessel, and nerve fiber in your body! It provides structural support and helps everything maintain its shape. You might have heard of myofascial massage, which helps loosen fascia around muscles, especially after injury or scar tissue formation.

Fascia is like a spider web—movement in one area can affect distant areas of the body. Imagine pulling a thread in a knitted sweater: one small tug can distort the entire shape! The same goes for your fascia—it's all connected.

Here's where it gets really interesting: the role of fascia in hydration has only recently been discovered. Until Dr. Jean-Claude Guimberteau's 2007 film, Strolling Under the Skin, fascia's importance wasn't fully understood. In fact, it wasn't until this film that we actually saw water being delivered to tissues via the fascia!

Fascia works like your body's own drip-irrigation system, delivering water to your tissues. While blood was once thought to be the primary carrier of hydration, we now know fascia plays a critical role. But here's the catch: fascia doesn't have a built-in pump, like the heart does for blood. It relies on movement to do its job.

So, exercise plays a huge role in detoxification and hydration!

I know, I can hear some groans out there. But don't worry—research shows that even "micro movements" like fidgeting can positively impact circulation and hydration. Remember the spider web analogy? Wiggling your toes or moving your foot can help hydrate your legs!

Gentle twisting motions are especially effective. Think of it like wringing out a towel to get the water moving. You can do simple torso twists in your chair right now. Not only will this stretch your muscles, but it will also hydrate your organs!

Easy movement exercises:

A great exercise to get your fascial hydration system going is the classic qi-gong arm-swinging exercise. Anyone can do it—no matter your age or fitness level! Here's a video to demonstrate:

https://youtube.com/shorts/SErWVZ_IAeY

Start by standing with your feet shoulder-width apart, knees soft, and gently swing your arms. Let them rise in front of you to shoulder height, then just let them drop and swing. You can add some gentle knee bends for good measure. Do this for a few minutes, or extend it into a 30-minute workout. You'll be surprised by how energized you feel from such a simple movement!

You can also try a similar arm-swinging exercise, but with a torso twist:

https://www.youtube.com/watch?v=
KyTroRUPnP0

Your Day 3 Homework

Set a timer for 25 minutes and spend that time moving your body. While you move, focus on how each motion brings precious hydration to your liver and other organs. Put on some music you love or an engaging audiobook and try the arm-swinging exercises while you listen. If it feels like too much, you can always lay down and do gentle pelvic tilts. Even wiggling around in your chair counts—every motion helps!

Give your liver a friendly pat, set your timer, and get moving!

Tomorrow, we'll learn how your liver is kind of like a bank... and how you can get out of overdraft!

~

4

DAY 4: THE LIVER BANK

I HOPE you're already starting to notice the benefits of better hydration. It might take some time, but you'll likely be amazed at how many physical and mental improvements can come from that one simple shift!

You may have noticed that I often ask you to set a timer for 25 minutes to complete tasks. Why 25 minutes? That unit of time is called a **Pomodoro**.

I first learned about the Pomodoro technique from Jim Kwik's book, *Limitless*. Jim is a world-renowned brain coach who overcame a severe brain injury as a child and became a master of optimizing mental performance. One key idea is that our brains remember beginnings and endings best—but not so much the middle.

You've probably noticed this yourself: you can easily recall the first person and the last person you meet at a party, but struggle with remembering everyone in between!

The Pomodoro technique leverages this by creating lots of beginnings and endings. It turns out that 25 minutes is the perfect time for our brains to focus without hitting that fuzzy "middle" zone. So, when you're doing a brain-intensive task—like reading, writing, or even today's liver challenge—break it into Pomodoros. Focus for 25 minutes, then rest for 5 minutes. Rinse and repeat. You'll be amazed at how much more you can get done!

Back to your liver!

You can think of your liver like a bank. It stores resources—like fat-soluble vitamins, minerals (such as copper and iron), and glycogen (a major energy source)—to be released when needed.

But let's think of our "liver bank" in terms of its overall capacity to do its many jobs. When your liver is struggling and you feel the need for a detox, it's a sign your "liver bank" might be in overdraft.

Just like with money, everyone starts with a different balance. Some people seem to have limitless reserves; they can party hard for years without seeming to suffer much for it. Others feel bloated after just one sip of wine! Genetics, early life factors (like mom's lifestyle during pregnancy), and past behavior all contribute to your starting balance.

But don't worry! No matter where you're starting from, you can build your reserves and get out of overdraft. The goal here isn't to take away everything you love, it's about balancing withdrawals and deposits. It's fine to make withdrawals, as long as your balance can handle it!

What counts as a "withdrawal" from your liver bank?

You probably know many of them already:

- alcohol
- sugar

- drugs and medications
- chemicals (absorbed through skin, air, food)
- infections
- allergies
- large meals
- processed foods
- deli meats
- holding onto grudges and chronic anger

And what about deposits? Here's how you can top up your liver bank:

+ dark leafy greens (like chard, beet greens, collards)
+ bitter foods (such as dandelion greens, bitter melon)
+ beets
+ aerobic exercise
+ fatty fish (salmon, sardines, tuna)
+ avocados
+ walnuts
+ garlic
+ green tea
+ coffee (unless you have adrenal overload)
+ good hydration
+ exercise
+ lean proteins (tofu, whey)
+ the attitude of gratitude

TODAY'S HOMEWORK

It's time to make your liver balance sheet! Set your timer for one 25-minute Pomodoro and grab a sheet of paper (or open a document). At the top, label it "My Liver Bank."

Start by writing your Starting Balance. How do you feel right now? If your liver balance were like a bank account, what would you estimate is in there? $10,000? $2,500? -$50? There's no right or wrong answer—just go with your gut.

Next, create two columns. Label one Deposits and the other Withdrawals.

On the left side, write down your "deposits"—the things you do that help your liver. Give them a value:

Ate a bowl of swiss chard: +$25

Did 45 minutes of cardio: +$100

Drank a quart of water: +$25

Ate a blueberry: +$0.50

Now, on the right side, list your "withdrawals":

Drank a glass of wine: -$20

Ate a pizza: -$50

Spray-painted in the garage without a mask: -$100

The values are arbitrary, but they'll help you reflect. What does your balance sheet look like? Does it match how you've been feeling? If it's heavy on withdrawals, think about how you can consciously start adding more deposits.

Just like with traction vs. dis-traction, ask yourself throughout the day: "Is this a deposit to or a withdrawal from my liver bank?" No judgment—just notice.

What did you discover when you wrote down your deposits and withdrawals? Feel free to send me a copy of your balance sheet if you'd like—but it's totally fine if you want to keep it private!

Tomorrow, we'll dive into one of the MOST important areas of detoxing without supplements or crazy diets: EMOTIONS!

Keep up the great work with your hydration, movement, and balance-checking habits!

My Liver Balance Sheet

Starting Balance:

Deposits	Withdraws	Balance

Ending Balance:

5

DAY 5: LIVER EMOTIONS?

THIS WAS ORIGINALLY DESIGNED as a 30-day detox challenge.

So why are we talking about emotions?

Well, when it comes to health, there are four big categories: structure, nutrition, toxicity, and emotions. Any health issue you can think of will show up in one or more of these areas.

When it comes to liver detoxing, we often focus on the chemical side—what we ingest, how toxic we become, and what we take to detox. But this isn't a sustainable long-term solution. That's why, in this challenge, we're working on the lesser-known aspects of liver health: structure and emotion.

Emotion is a biggie!

In fact, it can overshadow the other areas, influencing them in significant ways. In Chinese medicine, specific emotions are attributed to the liver. This might sound odd at first but think about it.

What are emotions, and how do you know you're having one? Emotions aren't just in your head, *they're in your body!*

For example, anger is closely linked to the liver. How do you know you're angry? You feel it physically—tension rises in your body, your jaw tightens, your heart races, and your blood rushes to your extremities, preparing you to fight. If you're feeling relaxed, muscles soft, and heart calm, you'd likely say you're not angry at all.

Fear, on the other hand, feels completely different: sweaty palms, shakiness, and the urge to shrink away. If you're scared enough, you might even have an accident! You get the idea.

These body-emotion connections aren't just in Chinese medicine—they show up in our language, too. Ever heard the phrase "galled"? It means shocked and angry, and it relates to the liver and gallbladder. Whoever came up with that word understood the connection between emotions and the organs.

So, what are the emotions tied to the liver?

They include:

- anger
- depression
- resentment
- frustration
- rage
- aggression
- emotional repression
- irritability
- indecision
- irrationality

In my entire career, I've never seen anyone with liver stress who didn't have challenges with these emotions. Think you might be the exception? Sorry, friend. You're not.

But don't worry—you don't have to "fix" your feelings. Emotions are just emotions. The goal here is to find balance and take some stress off the liver so you can feel better.

So, which came first? Did liver stress cause anger, depression, and indecision, or did those emotions cause liver stress? The truth is, it doesn't really matter. The body's nervous system is a two-way street. Causes and effects can ping-pong in either direction. Luckily, solutions work both ways, too.

I've seen many cases where improving the liver lifts emotions, and I've seen emotional healing help the liver recover. The body is amazing that way.

TODAY'S HOMEWORK

Take a close look at your life and identify what's making you angry, depressed, or frustrated—no judgment, just observation. Set a timer for 25 minutes and list the things that bring up these "liver emotions." If something makes you REALLY angry or upset, write it in all caps! Circle or underline the ones you feel strongest about, but keep writing for the full 25 minutes.

Think you're not that angry? Start small. It can be as tiny as your neighbor parking just close enough to your car to make it hard to open your door. Or maybe you're annoyed that your favorite jellybeans were missing from the bag. Anything goes—just find the things that stir a strong feeling and write them down.

This list is for your eyes only. You don't have to share it with anyone.

Since today is Day 5, you have the weekend off from new assignments! Use the time to finish anything you haven't yet completed. And if you're caught up, keep focusing on hydration, movement (even micromovements), and asking yourself if you're making deposits or withdrawals from your "liver bank."

Most importantly, resist the urge to judge yourself. Judging yourself won't help—it's just about noticing right now.

When you eat or drink, pay attention to the emotions that come up. Is there an emotion tied to eating something "good"? Or something "bad"? Just notice. You can jot them down if it helps, but the main goal is awareness.

Tomorrow, I'll show you a great way to neutralize some of these negative liver emotions. You —and your liver— will feel so much better. Give your liver a little pat and say, "We're going to feel a lot better soon!"

～

6

DAY 6: GRATITUDE

WELCOME TO DAY 6!

Are you already starting to feel better?

We ended last week by talking about "liver emotions," and how emotions like anger and depression can have a huge impact on your health.

Anger is uniquely harmful. While all emotions have their place, anger is the only emotion that's been scientifically shown to have strong negative effects on health. It can literally shorten your life! The system most harmed by long-term anger is your cardiovascular system.

For instance, in the two hours after an angry outburst, your chances of having a heart attack double. Anger also increases your risk of stroke, high blood pressure, lung problems, anxiety, and depression.

In fact, depression is often considered the flip side of anger. It's often described as anger turned inward.

So, what's the antidote to anger?

There's one emotion that's been shown to have the opposite effect on your body. A lot of people assume it's happiness. It's not. It's gratitude.

Gratitude has been scientifically proven to lower blood pressure, relax the heart rate, and improve breathing. In other words, it's a powerful counterbalance to anger.

But in our busy lives, we often forget to focus on gratitude, even though we all have a lot to be grateful for!

I experienced this firsthand in a strange way.

A few months ago, I had a profound shift in my gratitude levels after an unexpected few days of interacting with a scammer from The Gambia (a small country in West Africa) via Instagram Messenger. Long story!

Like all good scammers, he told me some things that were false, but many things turned out to be true. I had never even heard of The Gambia, so I researched it and listened to his stories. What started as skepticism turned into a profound shift in my perception of my own life. I realized I wasn't just "getting by"— I was living in absolute abundance. Suddenly, I felt blessed beyond belief and could see luxury in all the places where I'd been taking things for granted.

After cutting off contact with the scammer when he made his big move, I was left with this newfound gratitude. It went beyond material things—I felt grateful for my life, my kid, my friends, and even my city and country. I was so moved by the experience that I wanted to help people in The Gambia and found a reputable charity right here in Emeryville called Gambia Rising (www.gambiarising.org). They provide tuition for students, and the costs are incredibly low!

The point is, sometimes it just takes a shift in perspective to realize how much we have to be grateful for.

Today's exercise:

Your task today is to tap into the attitude of gratitude and hold onto it as much as possible throughout your day.

Some people can easily access that feeling, while others might need to work at it—especially if you're going through a tough time. Don't worry if it takes effort; it's worth it.

Set your timer for 25 minutes and simply list things you're grateful for. Don't worry about making the list long. It's more important to feel the emotion of gratitude than to fill up the page. And yes, you're allowed to be grateful for "bad" things, too! If something lights up that feeling of gratitude, it belongs on your list.

Anger is just a part of life.

It's inevitable that someone or something will make you angry at some point. And sometimes, anger is even justified. But the good news is, gratitude can neutralize the physical effects of anger on your body.

So today, give your liver a little pat and let it know you're grateful for it!

And try to carry that feeling of gratitude with you throughout the day.

~

7

DAY 7: SLOW IT DOWN

OK! It's Day 7, and even though emotions are huge, we're going to step away from them for a bit.

The most basic definition of toxicity is having something in your body that shouldn't be there—stuff like heavy metals, poisons, etc. That much is a no-brainer. But toxicity can also happen when there's too much of a good thing.

Did you know there's even such a thing as water intoxication? It happens when you drink too much water, and yes, it can actually be fatal!

The same is true for your liver. Sometimes, you're just giving it too much to handle.

Let me tell you a story.

I used to foster kittens for the SF/SPCA. When you foster kittens, you have to feed them very specific amounts of food. They need a lot of calories because they're growing, but you have to feed them in small amounts. Otherwise, they'll eat like crazy, digest very little, and leave you with messy, loose poops to clean up.

When they're eating, they're just sooooo cute—they want more food so badly, and it's hard to resist giving it to them! But after a few cleanups, you quickly learn to resist.

Aside from the mess, overfeeding is bad for their health.

Now, here's the thing: you're kind of like those kittens.

(And yes, you're adorable, too!)

But who's stopping you from overdoing it? Nobody! That's why you have to be the adult and slow down.

Are you always rushing to eat? If you've got kids, a job, or just a busy life, the answer is probably yes. But here's the problem: your digestive system—and your liver—don't work well under stress.

When your body perceives stress, it activates the fight-or-flight response. Blood and resources are diverted away from digestion to your muscles, preparing you to fight or run. Your brain doesn't know you're just rushing to pick up the kids or get back to a meeting. It thinks you're in danger, and digesting a meal is low on the priority list!

So how do you let your body know it's safe to eat and digest?

You breathe slowly and deeply, and you chew your food calmly and peacefully.

Marc David, the author of *Mind/Body Nutrition*, recommends taking 10 deep breaths before every meal. This calms your sympathetic nervous system (fight/flight) and lets your parasympathetic nervous system (rest/digest) take over so your body can focus on digestion.

I know 10 deep breaths can feel like forever. My monkey mind goes crazy when I try! But one day, I timed it. Guess how long it took me? A minute and a half.

I know you're busy, but do you think you can spare a minute and a half to let your body know it's OK to eat? And while you're eating, keep breathing deeply and chew slowly, like you have all the time in the world—even if you don't.

And if you don't finish by the time you "have to" go? Pack it up and save it for later.

Here's a crazy fact:

When you digest your food more efficiently, you won't need as much! Don't worry about getting enough food if you slow down. If you're reading this, you're probably getting enough.

Today's assignment:

You don't need to set a timer today (unless you want to time your breaths for fun!). Just take 10 deep breaths before eating anything, and then try to keep breathing deeply throughout your meal. If you don't finish your meal, no big deal—pack it up and see if you actually feel hungry later.

Now that you know how deep breathing can help your digestion and reduce toxicity, the idea of saying grace before meals takes on a whole new meaning!

Let me know how the deep breathing is going for you!

And don't forget to give your liver a little pat for all the hard work it's doing to help you detox.

～

8

DAY 8: ONLY THE BEST

OK! It's Day 8, and now we know that gratitude, slowing down, and even eating less all help to reduce the toxic load on the liver.

But you know what else can help? Only going for the BEST of your vices.

A good bad thing?

Sort of!

For example, let's say you're partly overstressing your liver due to a sugar habit. And let's say one of your sugar vices is chocolate. You can't pass the candy aisle without grabbing something, and gods help you when Halloween candy starts appearing on the shelves in August!

If chocolate is your vice, aim to only eat the BEST chocolate you can find.

For me, this means only buying from Christopher Elbow, an unbelievable luxury chocolate shop down the street. Their chocolate is otherworldly! But it's also spicey pricey. For the price of a 2-pound bag of Halloween chocolate, I can get maybe

4 small bonbons from Christopher Elbow! Needless to say, I'm not buying in bulk, and I'm not eating very much chocolate on any given day. Most days, I don't eat any at all.

But when I do eat it? It's heavenly! It almost makes me want to burst into song. (And if you know me... you know that's saying something!)

Whether your liver-stressing vice is pizza, wine, cheese, or chocolate, aim to stop it with the cheap, bulky stuff and only go for the best. Even if it means going a few days without, the experience will be totally different when you have it. You'll find yourself savoring it because it's harder to get and feels like a real treat!

Not only will you **naturally** eat or drink more slowly, but you'll get a better endorphin rush because it really is so much better than the cheap stuff. And you won't "miss" your old, daily or larger-sized indulgences because you'll look forward to these special moments of enjoyment!

Today's homework

Pick a daily (or almost daily) liver-stressing vice and commit to only getting the best version of it.

How do you know it's the best?

It usually feels a little uncomfortable to buy. Like, "Am I an idiot for paying this much for such a tiny portion? Is this really worth it?" It might feel strange to skip a few nights of dinner wine just to have that amazing "special occasion" wine on Friday. But trust me—it's worth it.

Remember the liver bank:

How much of a withdrawal is this vice?

Minus 5 bucks for the sugar in that fancy piece of candy?

Plus 30 bucks for the intense feeling of gratitude and satisfaction?

That's a net positive!

Now contrast that with a half-pound of Halloween candy:

Minus 30 bucks for the sugar, low-quality ingredients, chemicals, and sheer volume.

Emotional impact? Meh.

Definitely a net loss to the liver bank.

Which liver vice(s) will you commit to upgrade from a net loss to a net gain?

Give your liver a pat and let it know, "We're going to have a good time!"

∽

9
DAY 9: LESS IS MORE

OK, so a couple of days ago we talked about how toxicity can come from too much of a good thing, and we also talked about slowing down so your body can do the work of digesting.

You know another way to decrease the risk of overload?

Reducing the load.

Now before you get your panties in a bunch, I'm not suggesting you deprive yourself or starve yourself! We're just going to make a simple shift.

You've probably heard about SAD: the **S**tandard **A**merican **D**iet. And yes, it is sad. When we think of the SAD diet, we usually think about all the processed and refined foods, but that's not the only issue. It's the sheer volume that's also a problem.

As Americans, we're proud to live in a country where food is plentiful, and the portions are large. But what's so great about big portions? Unless you're doing manual labor—like construction or farm work—you're probably eating way more than your body needs!

Let me share a story.

A couple of years ago, some friends from Russia stayed with me for a few days during their whirlwind U.S. tour. I may be a world-class introvert, but I also take pride in being a great host (for up to 72 hours, max!). I wanted to make sure we ate well, so every time we stopped for food, I was ready to indulge in good stuff!

But I noticed something: they would only ever order tea and maybe split an appetizer or a small bowl of soup. At first, I thought they were just being thrifty travelers. By the second day, I finally asked if they were trying to save money.

They laughed and said, "No! We just can't believe how much food Americans eat!" They told me that American portions were too big and they wouldn't feel good if they ate that much at one meal.

When I tried to imagine shrinking my portions down to the size of what my Russian friends were eating, my brain resisted big time. I felt pushback—anger, even anxiety. These feelings were irrational, but they were real.

After they left, I decided to try out my own "Russian diet" for a month. All I did was cut my portions in half.

The results? I felt fine!

Physically, I felt good—lighter, more clear-headed. I even saved a lot of money! My food expenses were almost cut in half (I still had to buy food for my son half the time).

The only real resistance came from my mind. My mind panicked a little when it saw I wasn't going to eat the full meal. But when I checked in with my body, it felt perfectly fine. If I got hungry later, I ate.

TODAY'S HOMEWORK

Continue with the basics you've been practicing hydrating, moving, eating more slowly, and breathing deeply before meals...

And now, shrink your portion. Just cut it in half of whatever you would have eaten.

This isn't about dieting or deprivation. It's about discovering what your body really needs to feel good versus what you're doing out of habit.

Just pay attention. If you're hydrated, eating slowly, and breathing deeply, how do you feel after your half-meal? If you're still hungry, keep eating! But if you're not, and it's only your mind telling you to keep going, then stop. Wrap it up and save it for later. The next time you return to it, check in with your body again. Are you actually hungry, or are you eating just because it's there?

How did you do? Were you still hungry after the half-meal? Did you need your usual portion to feel satisfied?

Tomorrow, we'll do a great mindfulness exercise you can use in all areas of your life, not just for your liver!

Give your liver a little pat and let it know you love it!

~

10

DAY 10: MINDFULNESS

BY THIS POINT in the challenge, you've probably noticed that emotions are a big part of the journey.

Even when you're working on tasks that don't seem directly tied to emotions—like drinking more water or breathing deeply before meals—those emotions still show up! And often, they can get in the way.

One great way to bring intense, stressful emotions down a few notches is through mindfulness.

Here's a simple mindfulness exercise I learned from Dr. Nick Campos. It's incredibly powerful for helping to reduce the intensity of any stressful emotion by giving you a balanced perspective.

Here's how to do it:

Take a sheet of paper or open a blank document.

At the top, write down the problem or situation that's stressing you out.

For example: "I am going bald." (This caused me a lot of distress in the early days!)

Next, make four columns:

Column 1: "The worst thing about this problem."

Column 2: "The best thing about this problem."

Column 3: "The worst thing about if this problem didn't exist."

Column 4: "The best thing about if this problem didn't exist."

Now, write 20 things under each column.

If 20 feels too hard, start with 10, but you'll get more out of the exercise if you push for 20! And it's totally fine if some of your answers are ridiculous, as long as they're true for you.

For example, with my baldness problem, here's how the first few might look:

Worst thing: It accentuates my small, potato-shaped head.

Best thing: I'll save a ton of money on shampoo.

Worst thing if it didn't exist: I might've stayed a vain douche canoe with no compassion for bald guys.

Best thing if it didn't exist: I'd have continued to enjoy my cute hair.

Worst thing: I'll have an even harder time attracting a cute partner.

Best thing: I won't have to go to a hairdresser anymore.

Worst thing if it didn't exist: I would've had to keep seeing a hairdresser forever.

Best thing if it didn't exist: I'd still be networking with my hairdresser.

Why does this work?

Writing things out like this often reveals inner conflicts you didn't even realize you had. I had no idea I had so many mixed feelings about hairdressers until I did this exercise!

The goal of the exercise is to neutralize the emotional charge of whatever is stressing you out. Once you've written down so many pros and cons, the problem starts to feel less extreme— and therefore less stressful.

By seeing all sides of the issue, you give your mind a chance to find balance, which reduces emotional intensity and helps take pressure off your liver.

TODAY'S HOMEWORK

Set a timer for a Pomodoro session and try this mindfulness exercise for any problem that really stirs up major "liver emotions" for you. What's something that makes you really mad, depressed, or frustrated? Write it down and go through the columns.

Hit reply and let me know how you felt before versus after the exercise!

And don't forget to give your liver a little pat and let it know that it's all good!

Sample Mindfullness Worksheet

The Problem is:

Best Thing About this Problem	Worst Thing About this Problem	Best Thing if this Problem Did Not Exist	Worst Thing if this Problem Did Not Exist

11

DAY 11: UNDER PRESSURE

TODAY, we're talking pressure—acupressure!

I didn't think much about the power of pressure points until I met a special patient years ago who had basically healed herself of a rare liver disease. She told me that daily self-acupressure was a key part of her miraculous recovery.

Here's her story:

She was young—in her early 20s—and seemed healthy, but she had experienced a rare liver disease that destroyed most of the right lobe of her liver. Since the right lobe is the bigger one, she qualified for a transplant. However, there was no liver available, so she was put on the waitlist... a long list.

While waiting, she did everything she could to support the tiny part of her liver that was left: she worked on her diet, avoided sugar and alcohol, ate lots of vegetables, meditated, did yoga, and got chiropractic, acupuncture, and NET (which is how she ended up in my office).

Finally, she got the call—a liver was available! But when she went in for pre-transplant ultrasounds and lab work, there was a surprise. After about a year of intense liver self-care, her tiny left lobe had grown so large that it basically replaced the damaged right lobe! She no longer needed a transplant.

I had never seen results like that before, but her dedication to healing was beyond inspiring. And a big part of her routine was acupressure.

Now, I want to share some of those same liver-boosting acupressure points with you. These simple points can support your liver, help with detox, and even relieve some of those pesky "liver emotions."

The 7-Minute Liver Acupressure Routine:

LI-4 ("Adjoining Valley")

You probably already know this point—it's commonly used for headaches. This point is on the hand, in the web between the thumb and index finger. Liver stress often causes headaches, especially if you've consumed things like high-fructose corn syrup (I know, I avoid it like the plague because it triggers headaches for me within 20 minutes!).

To activate: Pinch or press toward the bone below the index finger for 90 seconds to 3 minutes. Start with 90 seconds if it's tender.

PC-6 ("Inner Pass")

This point is on the inside of the wrist, about three finger widths up from the base. It's not only great for liver health but also helps with nausea, motion sickness, and calming emotional stress.

To activate: Press the center of the inside of your wrist for about 2 minutes.

LV-3 ("Great Rushing")

This is a key liver point, and it might be tender if your liver is stressed. It's located on the top of the foot, in the web between the big toe and second toe. A massage therapist in Finland recommended this point to me, and it's powerful for moving stagnant liver energy.

To activate: Pinch with your hand or use a round object (like the back of a pen). You can also use the heel of your other foot while sitting at your desk!

LV-5 ("Woodworm Canal")

This point is located about a hand width above the inner ankle, just under the shinbone. It's a fantastic point for liver health and has the added benefit of boosting energy and helping with depression. It's even nicknamed "Liver 5 Alive!"

To activate: Hold for about 1 minute.

SP-6 ("Triple Yin Crossing")

This point is located three finger widths above the inner ankle. It supports not just the liver but also the kidney and spleen, making it a triple threat!

To activate: Hold for about 1 minute.

How do you feel after working on these liver points?

Were some of them tender? Do you feel more energized or more relaxed after working with them?

Hit reply and let me know how you felt after stimulating these liver-boosting acupressure points!

And give your liver a little pat and a rub, like it's your friendly dog. Who's a good liver?

p.s. I made a YouTube video demonstrating these points:

https://youtu.be/A4-W6SeLldw

~

12

DAY 12: CAN'T VERSUS DON'T

TODAY'S CHALLENGE is a simple one, but it's a game changer!

It's all about a small shift in language that can make a huge difference in how you feel about the foods, substances, or behaviors that stress your liver. Our words carry emotional weight, and that emotional weight can influence how we behave and how much stress we put on our liver.

It all comes down to two words: can't vs. don't.

When we say that we "can't" eat, drink, or do something, it usually comes with a negative feeling—like we're being deprived, or that we're not good enough for something. It's got emotional baggage.

For example, if someone offers you a cigarette, what do you say?

If you're a non-smoker, you simply say, "No thanks—I don't smoke." And that's it. It doesn't make you feel bad, and you don't feel like you're missing out on anything, right?

But if you were to say, "No, I can't smoke," it feels different. It's almost like you wish you could, but for some reason, you can't.

That little difference in language creates a totally different emotional response.

Now think about a fast, cleanse, or special diet. If someone offers you cake and you say, "No thanks—I can't," you might feel a little frustration, maybe some resentment, or even anger. (Hellooo, liver emotions!)

But if you're a vegetarian and someone offers you fried chicken, you simply say, "No thanks—I don't eat meat." It feels solid. There's no swirling emotion that could lead to a binge or a relapse. It's just a thing.

Today's challenge: Watch your language and practice saying, "I don't," rather than "I can't." This small shift will change how you feel about the choices you're making. Remember: of course, you can do whatever the hell you want! But you're choosing not to, because you don't do certain things.

Example responses:

"Is that all you're going to eat?"

"Yeah, I don't eat huge meals anymore."

"You don't want another drink?"

"Yeah, I don't. But thanks!"

This small habit shift can lead to a sense of empowerment and better results in many areas of your life—not just your liver health.

And when you indulge?

Say, "Yes, I'm doing that!" Own it.

And when you're not indulging, say, "No, I don't do that."

Don't be a sad sack with the "I can't."

This shift in language will help reduce frustration, anger, and all those "liver emotions" that can cause stress.

Hit reply and let me know how it feels when you switch from "can't" to "don't" in your language.

Give your liver a pat and say, "Thanks for helping me live a better life!"

∾

13

DAY 13: BREATH OF LIFE

ARE you surprised to find a day of breathing in a liver detox challenge?

Breathing is about more than just bringing in oxygen and getting rid of carbon dioxide! (Though oxygen is a super important part of detoxification.)

Deep breathing helps improve circulation and detoxification through the action of the diaphragm—a powerful muscle that we rarely think about since it's completely hidden from view! Plus, slow, deep breathing helps reduce blood pressure, which can be a big source of stress for your liver.

This reminds me of a story from one of my patients, a martial artist with years of Qigong experience (an ancient Chinese practice of meditation, controlled breathing, and movement exercises).

He was going through a health crisis and ended up in the ER. His blood pressure was sky high—180/150! They wanted to give him medication to lower it, but he didn't want any.

"Just give me a minute," he said.

He then settled in and started his Qigong breathing. Within minutes, he was able to bring his blood pressure back down to a healthy 120/80. His doctors were amazed.

While the story isn't meant to encourage anyone to ditch their meds, it shows how powerful breathing can be—even in extreme situations.

Breathing is a powerful addition to your supplement-free detox program!

And hey, you have to breathe anyway, right?

There are many different approaches to better breathing. The simplest is Mindful Breathing, *which just means paying attention to your breath.*

When you focus on your breathing, you'll naturally start to slow it down and take deeper breaths. Try to breathe from your belly instead of high up in your chest.

For today's breathing exercise, I want to introduce you to a phenomenal breathwork practitioner named Chuck McGee III. Chuck's story is pretty amazing. After facing major health challenges—he's a Type 1 Diabetic and a Traumatic Brain Injury survivor—Chuck was searching for ways to improve his health and stumbled upon breathwork. That's when everything changed for him.

He's traveled the world studying different breathwork methods, initially learning from some of the biggest names in the field, and now he's developed his own approach that's had a major impact on people struggling with chronic pain, anxiety, and depression. Chuck's goal is to empower people through breathwork that's tailored to their individual needs. One of the things I love about Chuck's work is that he acknowledges that no one-size-fits-all solution exists, and he's all about helping people find what works best for them.

Chuck does a free weekly breathwork session and Q&A via zoom. You can link to it through his website:

https://www.icedvikingbreathworks.com/
breathing-session

TODAY'S HOMEWORK

Mark your calendar and make sure to get to one of Chuck's breathwork zoom sessions!

In the meantime, add mindful breathing to your daily basics like hydration and slower eating.

And don't stress about it—remember, you're already breathing! Mindful breathing just means paying attention to your breath. If your brain starts wandering to worries or stress, gently guide it back by mentally saying the words "breathe in" whenever you are breathing in and "breathe out" whenever you are breathing out. Your brain can't easily think multiple thoughts or words at the same time, so by consciously thinking the words "breathe in" and "breathe out" with your breaths, it effectively blocks the brain from chattering about other things!

Bonus Challenge:

Take a moment right now to try a few mindful breaths. Breathe deeply from your belly and notice how it feels to give your diaphragm space to expand. Your diaphragm is right above your liver—imagine it giving your liver a little hug with each breath!

Tomorrow, we'll explore some more breathing techniques to help your liver thrive!

∾

14

DAY 14: BREATH OF LIFE (PART 2)

I SPLIT the breathing into two days because there are so many different approaches!

Yesterday, we focused on **Mindful Breathing** to help you get used to paying attention to your breath. Today, we'll explore a few other powerful breathing techniques that calm the mind, reduce stress, and support your body's natural detox processes.

Let's start with a simple but effective form of breathing: **Alternate Nostril Breathing**.

This technique calms the mind and reduces cardiovascular stress.

To do it, simply close one nostril with your finger and breathe in and out through the other. Then switch sides. Continue breathing slowly, alternating nostrils. This also stimulates both hemispheres of the brain, promoting balance and relaxation.

Many people use alternate nostril breathing before bed to settle the mind and body. Even just 5 minutes can lower your blood pressure and help prepare your body for deep rest.

Another yogic breathing technique is called **Ujjayi Breathing**, or "victorious breath."

This form of breathing detoxifies the body and mind and is also known as **ocean breath** due to the sound it makes.

To practice Ujjayi breathing:

1. Seal your lips and breathe in and out through your nose.
2. Take a slightly deeper inhalation than normal and exhale as slowly as possible through your nose.
3. As you exhale, constrict the muscles in the back of your throat to create a soft "ocean wave" sound.

This technique helps clear the mind, and the slow, deliberate breaths support detoxification by improving oxygen flow and circulation.

Next is the popular **4-7-8 Breathing**, which is based on Pranayama. Dr. Andrew Weil calls this technique a "natural tranquilizer for the nervous system." It's great for calming the body, especially during moments of stress.

Here's how to do 4-7-8 breathing:

1. Find a comfortable seat with your back straight.
2. Place your tongue against the back of your top teeth and keep it there.
3. Exhale completely through your mouth, making a whoosh sound.
4. Close your lips and inhale through your nose for a count of four.
5. Hold your breath for a count of seven.

6. Exhale completely through your mouth for a count of eight, making the whoosh sound again.
7. Repeat the cycle three more times.

This method helps regulate your nervous system and promotes deep relaxation. It's a powerful tool for reducing stress—one of the major contributors to liver overload!

TODAY'S HOMEWORK

Experiment with these breathing techniques throughout the day. Try them out when you're feeling stressed, or simply incorporate them into your routine to support detox and relaxation.

As you practice, think about any stressful situation in your life. Try one of the techniques and notice if it changes how you feel about that stressor.

Let me know which breathing exercise felt particularly helpful, or if you have a favorite I didn't mention! (In case you forgot, you can find me easily on LinkedIn!)

Give your liver a rub and a pat, and take a deep, slow breath.

∼

15

DAY 15: LIVER POSTURE?

I KNOW, I know... really?

Posture? For liver detox?

It's Day 15. Are we just making stuff up now?

Nope, it's true! The posture element actually pulls several things together. Sure, better posture has structural benefits, but the real power comes from the **neurological and emotional** benefits.

Did you know that there's a **negative liver posture**?

Think about it: what happens to your posture when you feel depressed, frustrated, or indecisive? You slump down, roll your shoulders forward, maybe frown.

Emotions affect posture—but it goes both ways! Your posture can also **affect your emotions**.

Do this experiment right now:

- Cross your arms.

- Slump down in your chair.
- Hang your head in a sad sack position.
- Put a frown on your face and furrow your eyebrows.
- Breathe shallow.

Now, try to think of the greatest day of your life! The happiest moment ever!

It's almost impossible to tap into that happy feeling while your body's stuck in that sad posture, right?

Now try the opposite:

- Sit or stand up straight.
- Shoulders back.
- Hands on your hips in the superhero position.
- Head slightly tilted up, with a big smile on your face.

Now, try thinking about the saddest day of your life. Really try to feel that awful feeling.

It's **almost impossible**, isn't it?

This posture trick shows how much our body language can influence our emotions and even our liver health. The more you sit up straight and adopt a **triumphant, open posture**, the better you'll feel emotionally—and the less stress on your liver!

What's your posture like when you eat?

For me, when a beautiful flan or tiramisu lands on my plate, I sit up straight, my face brightens, and if I had a tail, I'd be wagging it!

But if it's a plate of steamed greens? I notice I slouch a little. It's an unconscious habit—probably from childhood when bitter veggies meant dinner table battles.

What was your relationship to healthy foods when you were a kid?

Think specifically about foods that are good (or bad) for your liver.

What's your posture like when you're faced with these foods?

I'm not asking you to slump when you eat or drink something indulgent. But when you're eating or drinking something healthy, I am asking you to **sit up straight and proud**—in superhero posture!

Even if you're not craving that plate of bitter greens, adjusting your posture to an **open and cheerful one** while you eat can make the whole experience more positive. Your body responds to what your posture tells it!

By now, we know about the negative liver emotions.

But did you know there are also **positive liver emotions**? The main theme of the liver is **justice**. And what posture says "justice" better than **superhero** posture? Truth! Justice!

Today's homework

Pay attention to your posture when faced with healthy vs. unhealthy foods. Adopt a superhero stance when eating liver-friendly foods and notice how it changes your experience.

Did you have any revelations when you paid attention to your posture at meal times!

Sit up straight, shoulders back, head triumphant, and give your liver a pat. Let it know, "We're superheroes!"

～

16

DAY 16: POSITIVE LIVER EMOTIONS

SO FAR, **we've focused a lot on the "negative" liver emotions.**

Anger, resentment, frustration, depression, irrationality—these emotions can take a heavy toll on both your mind and your liver. But let's shift focus to the **positive** liver emotions today.

The positive emotions connected to the liver are:

- **Gratitude**
- **Forgiveness**
- **Patience**
- **Compassion**

The liver is often concerned with **themes of justice** and fairness. On the negative side, this can manifest as anger and resentment—the aggressive approach to justice. On the positive side, there's a more merciful approach, which involves compassion and forgiveness.

There's a time and place for both, but...

I wouldn't say both sides deserve equal time and energy in a happy and healthy life! If you can tip the scale toward **gratitude, compassion,** and **forgiveness**, you'll feel lighter and healthier—body, mind, and spirit.

Some people think of forgiveness as letting the other person off the hook. But forgiveness is really about **you**. It's about freeing yourself from carrying the toxic load of anger or resentment. You deserve peace of mind!

One of my mentors, Dr. Scott Walker, likes to say:

"The past is perfect. The future is up to us."

Anger and other negative liver emotions often come from **unmet expectations**. You expected something, and it didn't happen. The simple solution? **Let go of expectations.** The more you release expectations, the less you'll struggle with negative liver emotions.

Today's Exercise:

- **Set your timer for 25 minutes.**
- Write down everything that makes you really angry (or frustrated, resentful, etc.).
- Then, draw a line to see if you can connect each one to an **unmet expectation**—something you thought would happen but didn't.
- Next, see if you can shift your perspective. Is there a way to transform these feelings into **forgiveness, compassion**, or even **gratitude**?

Many successful people end up thanking their challenges. Malcolm Gladwell's book *David and Goliath* shows how disadvantages can turn into huge advantages.

You've already started practicing an **attitude of gratitude**. Can you expand it to include **compassion** and **forgiveness**?

How did you do? Was this exercise easy? Hard?

And hey, I know that some of you have been through really heinous things in life. I'm not saying you should "get over it" or forgive a monster who hurt you.

What I'm saying is that the **cost to your liver bank** is very high when it comes to holding on to negative liver emotions. Anger, resentment, and frustration take a toll.

I've seen it eat people alive.

So work on what you can—through breathing, mindfulness, movement—and make sure you have a trusted professional or friend to help you heal the deeper emotional stuff.

Give your liver a pat and let it know: "I'm grateful for you, and I have compassion for everything you've been through."

Tomorrow, I'll share a great tool to help move through some of those stubborn liver emotions!

～

17

DAY 17: FAST

MOST OF MY **career (since 1999) has been spent focusing on a mind-body healing method called Neuro Emotional Technique (NET).**

If you want to see a great example of NET in action, check out *Grey's Anatomy*, season 15, episode 22, "Head Over High Heels." In it, Owen tries NET for his PTSD and... spoiler alert —it works!

If you're encountering a lot of emotional resistance during this challenge, I recommend looking for an NET practitioner near you. You can find one at www.netmindbody.com, and if there's nobody near you, I work with people via Zoom for assisted FAST sessions.

But this challenge is all about **self-care**, so let's focus on what you can do for yourself!

Enter FAST

FAST stands for **F**irst **A**id **S**tress , and it's a quick, simple technique that came out of the NET world. You can find a video on how to do it at www.firstaidstresstool.com.

Here's the procedure in a nutshell:

1. **Identify an issue** that's stressing you out.
   - Example: Having way too many things on your plate and not enough hours in the day!
2. **Rate the intensity** of the stress on a scale of 1 to 10. Is it a 7? A 10?
3. **Place one wrist** (palm up) into your other hand. Using three fingers of your bottom hand, gently wrap your fingers around the wrist as if taking a pulse.
4. **Put your open palm** against your forehead, centering it between your eyebrows and hairline.
5. **Take a few deep breaths**, focusing on the feeling of the stressful issue.
6. **Switch hands** and repeat the process.
7. **Check in** with the intensity of the stress again. Where is it on the scale now? Did it drop down a notch? More than likely, it dropped down several notches!

Pro Tip: If you're dealing with **liver emotions**—like anger, frustration, or resentment—start with your **left wrist**, as this is where the specific liver pulse is located (middle of the three fingers). You might feel quicker relief!

One patient, recovering from a heart attack, brought along his friend, who was living in a tent encampment. The friend had chronic back pain, and though he wasn't looking for a handout, he asked if Medi-Cal could cover a visit. While they only allow two visits a month, I found that his back pain was actually **stress-related**.

After one visit, he felt a lot of relief, and I showed him how to do FAST Two weeks later, he came back and excitedly thanked me:

"Last week, someone pissed me off real bad, and I thought I was going to lose my mind! I was so mad I wanted to break something! But then I remembered that thing you taught me, and I did it, and all of a sudden, I wasn't mad anymore! I felt good! This shit really works! Thank you so much!"

In my perfect world, **FAST** would be taught in kindergarten! It's so simple yet so effective. People use it before bed, to help process the stress of the day. One 7-year-old patient even said it stopped her nightmares!

If you're feeling **toxic liver emotions** rising up, do FAST It really is fast!

And if FAST works well for you, you might love NET. Check out the documentary Stressed on YouTube to learn more:

https://youtu.be/ahU2FP_b9OQ

Let me know if FAST worked for you!

Give your liver a little pat and let it know, "We can feel better—FAST!"

THE HOMEOPATHY THING...

IF YOU READ through the F.A.S.T. website or look at the N.E.T. website, you'll see that they recommend homeopathy. This, for many "skeptical" people, is a dealbreaker. I get it.

Despite its widespread use in places like Germany—where it's covered by most health plans and frequently prescribed by medical doctors—there isn't a lot of scientific backing for it. And yet, despite the lack of hard evidence, 70% of patients report being very satisfied with homeopathic treatment. So what's that about?

I've been in practice long enough to know that **homeopathy does something**. I've seen it work on animals and babies, who wouldn't know the difference between a placebo and "real" medication. So, what's going on there? Honestly, I don't know.

I have a few theories as to why it may "work," even if Hahnemann's original theory of "like cures like" turns out to be false. One possibility is that it might be tapping into the body's natural ability to heal itself in ways we don't fully understand yet.

Whatever the mechanism, homeopathic remedies are so hyper-diluted that I firmly believe they do no harm. In the context of an N.E.T. treatment (or F.A.S.T.), they may take advantage of a principle called **state dependent learning**. This concept suggests that when the remedy is taken later, it can bring the body back to the state it was in during the original treatment, reinforcing the healing energy of that session.

There's a lot we still don't know about homeopathy—and healing in general. But just because we don't fully understand it doesn't mean it's not worth exploring.

Food for thought!

18

DAY 18: FIRE IT UP!

DURING THIS CHALLENGE, **we're going to cover two seemingly opposite concepts concerning the liver and "fire."**

One is about **supporting fire**, and the other is about **reducing heat**. Today, we'll focus on **supporting fire**.

What kind of fire?

In Chinese Medicine, the **Five Element Theory** groups all major organs into five elemental categories:

- **Earth**
- **Metal**
- **Wood**
- **Water**
- **Fire**

These elements interact with each other in different ways. For example, in one direction, each element feeds the next to help it grow. **Water supports Wood**, just like how staying hydrated supports liver health (the liver is in the Wood element!).

In the opposite direction, each element keeps another from becoming too intense. In this case, **Fire keeps Wood** (the liver) from growing out of control. When the liver is in a toxic state—overloaded and working too hard—it can benefit from the **balancing effects of the Fire element**.

What are the Fire element organs?

They include the **endocrine system**, the **cardiovascular system**, and the **small intestine**. People with liver toxicity often have weaknesses in these areas.

We've already talked about how eating more slowly helps the small intestine, and how movement—especially cardio—helps the heart. But what about the endocrine system?

The endocrine system includes the **adrenal glands**, which are crucial for regulating stress, metabolism, immune response, and blood pressure. The adrenals sit like little fatty hats on top of your kidneys, producing essential hormones to keep things in balance.

When the adrenals are weak, it's harder to keep the liver energy in check. Luckily, many of the things we've already covered—mindfulness, deep breathing, F.A.S.T., good sleep, slow eating—also help the adrenals!

Here are **two more** specific ways to support the adrenals and help them balance the liver:

1. Raw Sea Salt

Take a small pinch of unrefined sea salt (like Celtic Sea Salt or pink Himalayan salt) with your water a few times a day. This

can help the adrenals stay strong. Just avoid refined white table salt (umbrella girl salt), as it can raise blood pressure!
Bonus: A pinch of sea salt before bed can reduce nighttime trips to the bathroom.

2. Early Bedtime:
According to the **Chinese medicine body clock**, adrenal time is from **9-11 pm**. If you're in bed by 9 pm and ideally asleep by 10, your adrenals will get a much-needed boost. This also helps you sleep through **liver time** (1-3 am), which is when many people with liver issues wake up. Try going to bed earlier and see how much better you feel!

How does this support the liver?

By giving your adrenals the rest and support they need, you're helping your whole body—especially your liver—stay in balance. Strong adrenals prevent liver energy from becoming too intense, reducing stress on the liver and promoting better detoxification.

Let me know if you think your adrenals could use some support! (You can always find me on LinkedIn.)

Give your liver a pat and let it know, "Now we're cookin' with fire!"

∾

19

DAY 19: COOL IT DOWN

TOTALLY SEPARATE FROM the elemental Fire in the 5-element system, there's a concept of "heat" in Chinese medicine that basically means inflammation.

I mean, "inflamed" literally means "on fire," sooo... makes sense!

When the liver is stressed with excess toxicity, there's almost always inflammation. From the Chinese medicine perspective, this means there's **too much heat** in the liver!

What's the solution?

To counter this heat, you can focus on **cooling foods** and avoid things that bring in more heat. Some of this is intuitive—spicy or hot (temperature) foods can add heat to the liver. Seems legit.

But some cooling foods aren't as obvious. For example, **artichokes** are great for removing excess liver heat. Why?

Why not!

Here's a list of foods traditionally used to help combat liver heat:

- Seaweed
- Spinach
- Chestnut
- Rye
- Vinegar
- Asparagus
- Artichoke
- Egg
- Royal jelly
- Aloe leaf (dried juice concentrate)
- Bitter melon
- Burdock root
- Celery
- Dandelion greens
- Lemon
- Peppermint
- Tomato
- Water chestnut
- Zucchini

Don't you hate it when people throw a big list at you and expect you to remember it all?!

Don't worry—you don't have to memorize this list!

Part of this 30-day challenge is to give you **lots of tools** to help support your liver. You don't need to implement everything. You just have to find the most powerful, useful pieces that help **YOU** the most.

Remember Pareto's Principle?

80% of your results come from 20% of your efforts.

So what's your most powerful 20%? It's different for everyone, but keep your eye out for it and enjoy the ride!

Let me know which **liver-cooling food(s)** you can painlessly increase in your diet!

Give your liver a pat and tell it, "Cool it, friend. We're doing good!"

Tomorrow, we meet **Fletcher**.

~

A WORD ABOUT KITCHEN GEAR

THIS 30-DAY CHALLENGE **doesn't get into specific dietary regimens.**

But one of the biggest contributors to liver dysfunction in America is the increasing reliance on **processed and packaged foods**. Many of the packaged foods we consume contain ingredients that no one would have in their home kitchen! And guess who has to process all that stuff? Yep—your liver.

One simple way to take the pressure off your liver is to prepare more of your own food at home!

But... if you're "challenged" like me in that way ("a terrible cook"), well... that can feel rough.

For my fellow **culinarily-challenged** people out there, I recommend two quality pieces of kitchen gear to make it easier:

1. **A good strong blender**
   - This makes it easy to pulverize greens into healthy smoothies. Sometimes, it's just easier to drink your food than chew it all up!
   - When shopping for a blender, look for one with **high power** (at least 1000 watts) and **durability** to handle leafy greens and frozen fruit.
2. **An Instant Pot**
   - I was going to write about the **three** essential pieces of kitchen gear until I realized the Instant Pot does double duty as both a **pressure cooker** and a **slow cooker**!
   - Slow cookers are great for set-it-and-forget-it meals. Just throw in the ingredients, come back in a few hours, and boom—dinner is ready!
   - The pressure cooker setting, on the other hand, is perfect for quickly cooking healthy things (like artichokes) that usually take forever the old way.

If I can do it, so can you!

Supporting your liver doesn't have to be compli-cated. It starts with a few simple changes in the kitchen.

DAY 20: FLETCHERIZE IT!

I HAVE TO ADMIT, **I'm fascinated by the characters of the 19th century.**

It was such a wild time, right on the cusp of the technological boom of the 20th century! People knew something big was coming, but they didn't know what, so they hypothesized in all directions.

Sometimes, they hit on something true and timeless.

Sometimes, they were way off the mark.

Even so, there's often a kernel of truth even in the craziest of fads and fantasies.

One of the colorful characters of the 19th century was health faddist **Horace Fletcher**, known as **"The Great Masticator."**

His tagline?

"Nature will castigate those who don't masticate."

Fletcher developed stomach trouble and obesity later in life and went on a quest to find a solution. His extreme approach was **chewing**.

And by extreme, I mean he chewed his food beyond the point of liquification—until it lost its taste!

That... was probably too much. But!

There was some truth in his theory about the connection between health and chewing. It's true that most of us don't chew our food enough.

Remember how we talked about toxicity building up when there's too much for the body to handle?

Inadequate chewing burdens the liver in two ways:

1. Swallowing large chunks of under-chewed food makes digestion harder, putting more stress on your system.
2. Because the food isn't broken down well, your body doesn't absorb as many nutrients, leading to deficiencies. And then you need a bunch of supplements to fill the gaps!

Studies show that blending your food (like with smoothies) can increase nutrient absorption by up to **90%**! Can you imagine getting **nine times** the nutrition from the food you're already eating?

While it's not practical to blend all of your meals, **chewing more thoroughly** can have a similar benefit.

What if you could absorb just 40% more nutrients by chewing mindfully?

You'd be able to eat less but gain more nutrition! It's like magic.

Fletcher's followers recommended chewing each mouthful **25 times**, and the extreme chewers went up to **100**!

I can't even get to 25, to be honest—it's kind of gross. But when I paid attention, I found I was only chewing **2 or 3 times** before swallowing. That's too extreme in the other direction!

So start with **mindfulness**.

How many times are you chewing each bite of food?

Can you slow down, chew more thoroughly, and swallow something that will be easy for your body—and your liver—to digest?

Eating quickly and barely chewing is likely a byproduct of our abundant times, where food is readily available. When food is scarce, people tend to eat more slowly and mindfully.

So slow down, chew thoughtfully, and bring in that attitude of gratitude.

Give your liver a pat and give thanks for living in such an abundant time, especially when it comes to food. And imagine your body absorbing all the **beneficial nutrients** that your food has to offer!

Next week, we're going to get into the weeds!

～

BONUS THOUGHTS

IS EATING LIVER GOOD **FOR** YOUR LIVER?

Let's get one thing out of the way.

A lot of people believe the liver "stores" toxins. It **does not store toxins**! So, you're not "eating toxins" when you eat liver. (Well, no more than you would from eating any other part of an animal, depending on its overall toxicity status...)

In terms of nutrients, **liver** is an excellent source of **vitamin A** and a good source of **vitamins B** and **C**, as well as niacin, riboflavin, folate, iron, potassium, copper, and phosphorus.

You may notice that a lot of **liver support supplements** contain liver extracts. This stems from a nutritional theory that using **glandular extracts** supports the health of the corresponding organs. For example, a **pancreas support supplement** will contain pancreas, a **heart support supplement** will contain heart, and so on. The idea is that these tissues contain more than just nutrients—they may also contain **specific enzymes, hormones,** and **hormone precursors** that specifically support the organ in question.

There's plenty of **anecdotal evidence** and case studies suggesting this approach works. However, I'm not sure about any hardcore clinical studies proving it definitively.

Conclusion?

Can't hurt, might help!

21

DAY 21: STOP THE PRESSES!

STOP THE PRESSES!

Well, really, stop the eating... at a certain time...

I just really like saying "stop the presses!"

Today's lesson is **super short** and simple, but that's because it's so **singularly important**! I hope it sticks with you.

Remember the **Pareto Principle**? Where 80% of your results come from 20% of your actions?

Some practitioners say that, when it comes to **liver and gall-bladder health**, these two habits alone are **"80 percenters"**—they give you massive bang for your buck:

1. Stop eating 2-3 hours before bed.
Late-night eating creates **stagnation** in the liver, making it harder for the liver to do its nightly job of **cleaning and repairing** your body.

I'm not going to judge you [today] for what time you go to bed!

But whatever time it is, **stop eating 2-3 hours** before then.

2. Stop eating when you're about 80% full.

This means you're **kind of full** but could still eat more.
Just **don't**.

Eating until you're 80% full is a way to avoid **overloading** the liver and digestive system. It also gives your liver a break from constantly having to process a heavy load, allowing it to function more efficiently.

It's OK to feel a little uncomfortable!

Part of what we're learning with our increased **mindfulness** is to be OK even when we're a little uncomfortable.

It's pretty amazing how learning to tolerate a bit of **physical discomfort** makes it easier to handle **emotional discomfort** too.

And when you're able to tolerate feeling uncomfortable, what happens?

It becomes easier to get out of your comfort zone. And what happens when you do that?

NEW AND GOOD STUFF!

Have you ever been so excited about feeling a little uncomfortable!?

Give your liver a little pat and just smile and say, "ohhh, yeah."

22

DAY 22: BEET IT!

IT SEEMS like most supplements and products designed to cleanse the liver contain **beets**.

Why?

Well, I could list the 80-something nutrients found in beets, but that would be totally meaningless!

It'd look like, blah-blah-blah-blah-6-blahblah-12-blah-blah-blah...

Just know that **beets** are darn good for your liver (and your gallbladder).

And the **greens** are just as good!

Once, someone at a farmer's market sold me a huge bag of beet greens for like $1 because he was about to throw them away! Most people wanted the beets without the greens.

I get it. The greens are kind of **bitter** and **tough**, and they're not much to look at.

But cook them up and you'll feel better in your body than you expected! You can almost feel the soothing effect on your **liver** and your **mood**.

Beets and beet greens are like **$50 bills** to your liver bank.

If you have a choice between healthy options, go for beets and their greens. For example, kale is popular and healthy, but when it comes to liver health, a kale salad is like a $30 deposit into the liver bank, while beet greens are like $50.

Even **chard** is almost as good! That's because chard is in the **beet family**. It's like a beet that was bred to have big, juicy leaves instead of a fat root.

Here's a simple **medicinal beet slaw** recipe that some people use as a gentle liver and gallbladder cleanse:

- **1 cup of shredded raw beets**
- **2 tablespoons of flaxseed oil**
- **Juice from 1/2 a lemon**

The **simple version**: take **2 tablespoons** of the mix **twice a day** for 1-4 weeks, along with some fiber if your diet needs it.

The **complex version**: take **1 teaspoon every 1-2 hours** for 3 days, then **2 tablespoons 3 times a day** for 7 days, and finally **2 tablespoons twice a day** for 4-32 days.

For most people with jobs and kids, that complex version probably won't happen. Just eat more **beets**—and don't forget the **greens**!

Did you know there are **other beet varieties** besides red? Some beets are **orange**, **rainbow-colored**, or even **white**.

White beets have a mild flavor, but unfortunately, they're missing the liver-healing component **betalain**, which gives red beets their color and helps the liver detoxify.

Pro-tip: Don't be alarmed if your pee and poop turn purple/red after eating beets! It can be freaky, but it's totally normal.

Do you think you can eat more beets?

If you hate beets, how about trying the greens?

Can **crystals** heal your liver??

Tune in tomorrow to find out...!

〜

EASIEST TASTY GREEN SMOOTHIE

WE ALL KNOW that the liver loves dark leafy greens. And we know that smoothies are a great way to get those greens in! But smoothies are such a pain to make. Do you need to remember to freeze stuff? Add fancy powders? A little o' this, a little o' that?

I love this one because other than water, it only calls for 3 ingredients, and it tastes great!

Ingredients:

1 small bunch of spinach

1 pear

Some fresh mint leaves

Put 'em all into a blender.

Add water to make it an acceptable consistency for you.

Drink!

. . .

That's it!

If only all healthy tasties were that easy. *sigh*

DAY 23: THE DARK CRYSTAL

(This chapter isn't really about *The Dark Crystal*. I just loved that movie when I was little and wanted to throw it in here because... today's topic is crystals!)

YOU MIGHT BE REALLY EXCITED to see this message about **crystals**!

Or... you might be a little disappointed in me.

But what can I say?

I love me some **crystals**.

Basically, I just love **rocks**.

They're amazing.

An introvert's best friend!

But let's get down to business.

Is there any legitimacy to **crystal healing**, and can it help you detox your liver?

Well, **yes and no**.

Mostly **"no"** in the metaphysical shop sense.

Sorry, but just because **bloodstone** looks like a liver—dark green like bile, with red like blood—doesn't mean that wearing it or sleeping with it under your pillow will magically detoxify your liver!

That said, there are rocks and crystals with legit physical properties.

After all, **salt** is a crystal rock.

Sulfur can be a rock.

And **tourmaline** is used industrially for its ability to absorb negative ions!

But more importantly, rocks and crystals can evoke **feelings** and serve as **reminders** to stay on track.

By now, you know—REALLY know—what a huge role **thoughts**, **feelings**, and **emotions** play in your liver health!

If a crystal can serve as a reminder and bring on a positive feeling, then **go for it**!

Think of it like wearing a **cross** around your neck. It reminds people of their values and helps guide them through life. (As opposed to... repelling vampires! Which, honestly, is what I thought crosses were for when I was a kid.)

Where your attention goes, energy flows.

What you focus on is what grows.

And in a world filled with distractions, we need every tool we can get to stay focused! So, if **crystals** make you happy and help you focus, then **use them**. They're a legit tool for bringing attention back to your goals.

Whether it's a bracelet or a ring made with stones that have traditional healing meanings, it can serve as a tangible, fun reminder to stay on track—way more interesting than a digital to-do list!

The more senses you involve in achieving your health goals, the better.

My favorite rocks are **sugilite**, **larimar**, and **ametrine**. But I also love **lapis lazuli**, **fluorite**, **rhodonite**, and **chiastolite**... OK, maybe they don't help me focus, after all!

Let me know if you find it helpful to have something solid to touch or hold that reminds you of your health goals.

Tomorrow, we'll be getting into a **bitter truth**...

∾

SHOULD YOU EVER PUT A CRYSTAL WHERE THE SUN DON'T SHINE?

The official answer is: **"No, Gwyneth. You shouldn't."**

But, being the kind of person I am—someone who just **has to know** from personal experience—I can neither confirm nor deny whether or not I've attempted such a thing!

During my weird "crystal phase," I tried it all. When it came to liver stuff, yes, I even taped certain rocks and crystals right over my liver area to see if I could feel any changes! I slept with specific rocks under my pillow, placed them in strategic spots around my room, and kept a giant chunk of **selenite** under my treatment table at the office. You know, to **"absorb negative energy."**

Why do I share these stories? So you know there's **no shame** here. If you've tried or are thinking about trying something a little "out there," feel free to ask me about it! Chances are, I've probably been there, done that. **I don't judge.**

Once, I had a terrible migraine and, in a moment of desperation, started massaging my head with a **fluorite wand**. Within minutes, the headache was gone! I had a couple more successes with the fluorite, but after that, the magic stopped. Was it really the rock that made the headache go away? Or was it something else? Now, every time I look at fluorite, I wonder, **"Did you really stop my headache?"**

But hey, if something brings you comfort—or even just a good chuckle in this often grim world—that's **good enough** in my book!

24

DAY 24: THE BITTER TRUTH

TODAY, we're talking about a bitter truth. The truth is...

Bitter foods are **really** good for your liver!!!

It's true. Just as sweet foods are often blamed for stressing out your liver, bitter foods can be the **antidote**.

Bitter is one of the tastes that's missing from the American diet!

The main place I can think of where it's regularly used is in the world of cocktails. And, you know, its benefits in that arena are probably...diluted by, well, the cocktail.

But here's the thing: the components that make foods bitter are often the same powerful protective substances that keep a plant safe from being eaten all the time. For us, they stimulate digestion and bile production, which is great news for our livers!

You don't have to go all out, though. I once tried to eat a whole bowl of salad made from just dandelion greens.

Too bitter!

I also once tried to eat a whole bitter melon. It did great things for my blood sugar and made me feel good emotionally afterward, but the eating part was, well...

TOO bitter!

So, don't be a weirdo.

It's totally fine to use moderation!

You can start small:

- Add some dandelion greens to your salad.
- Sauté some bitter melon with your eggs.
- Try adding Swedish Bitters to your water.

Start noticing the presence (or absence) of bitter flavors in your diet. Where can you bring them in? How could it be fun? Maybe even start a little "bitters kit" like my brother's Tapatio stash—he carries his own mini hot sauce just in case a restaurant doesn't have any. You could carry a little bottle of Swedish Bitters with you!

Swedish Bitters is an herbal tonic that's been used since the 15th century! It's known to relieve indigestion, gas, bloating, constipation, and improve nutrient absorption. Sound familiar? Yes, indeed, they're all things connected to **liver function**!

Bitter foods are big deposits to the liver bank.

Let me know if you already have some bitter foods or drinks you enjoy!

Give your liver a pat and let it know, "We're going to eat some bitter so we don't have to BE bitter!"

Tomorrow, I'm going to tell you about some **free bitters** that are probably sitting in your own backyard right now!

25

DAY 25: BACKYARD BOUNTY

RIGHT NOW, at this very moment, you probably have some powerful liver-detoxing foods growing in your own backyard!

(Well... if you have a backyard...)

You already know that dandelion greens are bitter and great for the liver. And yes, that includes those little dandelions growing in your yard! As long as the yard hasn't been sprayed with chemicals, those dandelions are totally edible.

If you've ever purchased a "detox tea" from the health food store or liver detox supplements, you'll notice that dandelion root is a common ingredient! You can harness the same benefits from the whole plant—leaves, flowers, and roots—right from your yard. Here's a great website that shares ways you can enjoy dandelions:

https://foodprint.org/blog/how-to-eat-dandelions/

Milk thistle is another common ingredient in liver detox products. In fact, an extract from milk thistle is even used in hospitals to combat mushroom poisoning!

But did you know that **all thistles** (in the genus *Cirsium* and *Carduus*) are edible?

That means if you find a thistle plant in your yard, it's not just a prickly nuisance—it's a nutritional powerhouse!

Thistles are packed with nutrients and are great for the liver. Here's more info on how to prepare and enjoy them:

https://eattheplanet.org/thistle-nutritious-and-beautiful-on-the-inside/

I'll be honest, though—I'm a terrible cook and pretty lazy in the kitchen.

So, my favorite way to prepare thistles is to toss them into my Ninja with other ingredients and blend the hell out of it! The blender safely obliterates the spines and unlocks all that nutrient goodness.

And my **#1 favorite bitter backyard plant of all**: Plantain weed!

(I have no idea why it's called plantain, and no, it's not related to the banana-looking thing!)

You've probably seen this plant around. It's super common! Here's a picture and more info about it:

https://gardenculturemagazine.com/plantain-the-overlooked-medicinal-weed/

You can toss the young leaves into a salad, sauté the older leaves, or even cook the seed stalks in butter. Plantain leaves are bitter, but they pack a big punch when it comes to liver health. I can literally feel the positive effects in my body when I eat them—especially a lift in mood that chases away that cranky, livery feeling.

. . .

Aside from being **free medicine**, foraging for your own food is a great way to slow down and be present. It's like a micro-vacation from the fast-paced modern world, and it gives you a sense of control over an important part of your health.

But always be cautious when foraging—make sure you properly identify the plants, and if you're unsure, don't eat them!

Here in the Bay Area, we're lucky to have a fantastic foraging book made just for us: *The Bay Area Forager: Your Guide to Edible Wild Plants of the San Francisco Bay Area* by Mia Andler and Kevin Feinstein. Kevin also teaches great foraging classes through foragesf.com, both online and in person.

Wherever you are, start simple! Why not toss a few dandelion or plantain leaves into your salad? It's free money for your liver bank!

Give your liver a pat and take it for a walk outside!

∽

ARE COFFEE ENEMAS REALLY GOOD FOR YOUR LIVER?

Apparently, soldiers given opiate painkillers often suffered from constipation, and enemas were a common solution. However, clean water was in short supply, so someone suggested using the day-old leftover coffee.

To everyone's surprise, patients who received the coffee enemas seemed to recover better than those who were given plain water enemas! It was postulated that the caffeine dilated the blood vessels around the liver, helping speed detoxification and support healing.

Is this story true? Probably not.

Coffee enemas were indeed used during the war, but it was actually by the Germans and as part of an anti-shock and anti-poisoning treatment. Unfortunately, it didn't turn out to be very effective, and the practice was eventually removed from medical manuals.

Nevertheless, coffee enemas took off in the world of alternative therapies, which of course meant that young me had to try it.

Because that's what I do!

Shortly after trying it, I felt weird, buzzy energy, and my heart started racing like I had just downed an entire pot of coffee.

Oh wait—maybe because I did?

Only this time, through my butt!

Needless to say, I didn't sleep well at all that night, and I'm just grateful my heart didn't explode.

Conclusion?

There are probably better things you could be doing for your liver.

I don't recommend coffee enemas—unless coffee gives you heartburn, and you're just looking for another way to get your fix!

26

DAY 26: ALLERGENS

WELL, here we are— the final week!

Are you keeping up with your hydration?

Breathing?

Slower eating?

Movement?

Attitude of gratitude?

And, of course, your general mindfulness?

I hope you're becoming more conscious of how the little things add up!

Today, we're talking about allergens.

When I say "allergens," I'm referring to things that aren't pathogens (like viruses or bacteria) but still trigger an immune response in the body—things like food, pollen, or dust.

Whenever your body detects something it doesn't want inside, your immune system kicks in. And, naturally, your liver is part of the cleanup crew!

For bigger culprits like dust and pollen, you can reduce your exposure with simple measures—like wearing a mask during yard work or when cleaning out dusty areas. (I think we all have masks.) Vacuuming under your bed helps too! I finally got a Roomba, and now my under-bed is delightfully dust-free!

But one of the biggest ways to ease the stress on your liver is by reducing or eliminating food allergens.

How can you test for food sensitivities?

Blood tests are the gold standard, but if you're on a budget, here's an easy DIY option:

Take your pulse before eating. Then, about 10 minutes after eating, check it again. If your pulse jumps by more than 10 beats per minute, you might have a sensitivity to that food.

You can also try this *low-tech* version of muscle testing:

Take a few deep breaths, paying attention to how they feel. Hold the food or drink close to your chest and, if possible, inhale its aroma. Then check your breath—has it become shallower or more constricted? That could be your body signaling a "no." If your breath feels more open or expansive, the food may be "good" for you.

· · ·

Be careful though—muscle testing isn't a "truth machine."

It's just a tool. There are many reasons why your body might respond to a certain food—sometimes it's purely emotional!

In the NET world, we sometimes treat "emotional allergies"— those physiological reactions triggered by unresolved emotions. For example, in his 1943 book *Release From Nervous Tension,*

Dr. David Harold Fink describes a patient with a severe rose allergy. One day, Dr. Fink placed a huge bouquet of artificial roses in his office. The patient immediately had a full-on allergic reaction—despite the flowers being fake! The issue turned out to be emotional, and once that was treated, the allergies disappeared.

So, if you notice your body reacting negatively to a food— whether through pulse testing, breathwork, or muscle testing— work on reducing or eliminating it from your diet.

Over time, as your body becomes healthier, it naturally becomes more resilient and less reactive to allergens.

Let me know what you discover when you try the pulse or breath tests!

Tomorrow, we'll dive into the topic of oils and fats.

Give your liver a hug and remind it that it's pretty awesome.

~

27

DAY 27: OIL IT UP

I WAITED until now to bring up the topic of oils because this challenge is about taking stress off of your liver without relying on supplements or crazy diets. Sometimes food information can feel overwhelming! But the truth is, oils are important, especially if you've been diagnosed with something like non-alcoholic fatty liver and are wondering if eating more fats will make it worse.

Healthy fats and oils are essential.

Not only do they help stimulate bile flow (keeping the bile ducts healthy), but they're crucial for:

- Absorbing fat-soluble vitamins
- Providing energy
- Producing hormones

But the type of oil you use in cooking makes a huge difference!

Here are some **"bad"** oils that can increase inflammation over time:

- Canola
- Cottonseed
- Corn
- Grapeseed
- Soy
- Safflower
- Rice bran
- "Vegetable" oil* (which is usually a blend of canola, corn, soybean, safflower, and other oils)

Now for the **"good"** oils that support health:

- Extra virgin olive oil
- Avocado oil
- Sesame oil
- Coconut oil
- Peanut oil
- Walnut oil
- Flaxseed oil

When cooking, make sure to check the **smoke point** for each oil. Some are great for high heat, while others (like flaxseed oil) are better suited for cold dishes, like salad dressings and smoothies.

Personally, I'm also a fan of butter and ghee, although some people may disagree.

I know healthy oils can be more expensive, but:

1. **It's worth it**
2. **You can afford it now** because you're eating less and absorbing more nutrients thanks to your mindful eating!

Remember, "saving money" on cheap, unhealthy oils can cost more in the long run—both in health expenses and in quality of life (and possibly even lifespan!).

About supplements:

Most Americans would benefit from an omega-3 supplement like fish oil, flaxseed oil, or black currant seed oil. The reality is, our diet and lifestyle choices often lead to inflammation, making these supplements helpful for reducing damage.

Hey, no judgment—I'm an American, too.

Been there, done that, got the t-shirt.

The key is to **stay mindful** and recognize that healthy oils are investments in your liver bank!

But listen, if you have a favorite recipe that uses some ungodly oil (like Granny's Crisco-slathered recipe), don't worry too much. That's a withdrawal from the liver bank. If the joy it brings you makes it a net deposit in your happiness account, go for it! Life's complicated, and **so are you.** And that's awesome.

Give your liver a pat and say, "You're complicated, and that's awesome."

Tomorrow, we're talking about your skin.

We're on the home stretch!

~

28

DAY 28: SKIN DEEP

SKIN HEALTH IS CLOSELY TIED to liver health.

Whenever someone comes in with skin complaints, the first thing I think is, "What's going on with the liver?"

In fact, if you've been doing your homework and keeping up with the basics over the past month, you've probably noticed your skin looking and feeling better—even if there was nothing "wrong" with it to begin with!

Remember how the nervous system works both ways?

Just as giving your liver some love will help your skin, giving your skin some extra love can help your liver, too.

How? There are two main ways:

1. **Moisturize, Moisturize, Moisturize!**

(RuPaul knows best!)

A good quality moisturizer isn't just great for your skin, especially as we get older.

Here's something that might surprise you:

A recent study suggested that regular use of moisturizer can help prevent dementia.

I know, it sounds like complete b.s.—until you check the fine print.

It's now known that chronic inflammation is a key factor that can lead to dementia.

Since inflammation is the all-around bad guy in so many health issues (including liver stress!), anything that reduces inflammation is a win.

Moisturizer??

Yes! It's because your skin covers such a large surface area, that reducing inflammation there has a significant effect on your overall body inflammation levels. Lower inflammation = less work for your liver!

Just make sure you're using a good-quality moisturizer that's free from harsh chemicals or synthetic fragrances, which can be counterproductive for your liver.

2. Skin Brushing: Detox for the Win!

Skin brushing is exactly what it sounds like.

Grab a soft-bristle body brush and gently brush your skin in the direction of your heart.

This does more than just exfoliate! It stimulates your lymphatic system, which plays a major role in detoxification.

The lymph system doesn't have its own pumping mechanism and relies on muscle movement to keep things flowing. If you're not getting enough movement, skin brushing can give your lymph system the extra boost it needs to help your body clear out toxins—taking some stress off your liver in the process!

So, give yourself permission to make time for moisturizing and skin brushing.

It's not just for vanity (though, why not?)—it's for your health!

Hit reply and let me know how skin brushing felt if you tried it!

Do you already have a go-to moisturizer that you love?

Give your liver a pat and let it know, "We're going to the mini-spa!"

Tomorrow, we're tackling the bullet you thought you dodged: sugar (and alcohol).

Stay tuned!

~

WHY ARE THEY CALLED "LIVER SPOTS" ANYWAY?

If you are a light-skinned person, you may start to develop brownish spots on your skin as you age. You may know them as "age spots" or "liver spots." (My doctor recently tried to make me feel better by calling one of them a "wisdom spot." Thanks, Doc, that helps.) So, why are they called "liver spots?"

Back in the old days, they were thought to be caused by liver problems, because they were basically the color of the liver: dark reddish or brown.

Nowadays, we know that they are really caused by prolonged exposure to the sun. They are made of melanin, which is what gives your skin pigment. Exposure to UV light increases melanin production, which is how you get a suntan! It's also how you get sunburns and sun damage!

Liver spots will tend to appear on areas that have been sunburned in the past or which have received a lot of sun exposure over time. That is why they are also called sunspots or solar lentigines. The best way to prevent them is to get a time machine and use lots of sunblock (at least SFP 30) and caution while you are young!

There is evidence that they can be made worse by ingestion of rancid oils, deficiency of certain vitamins such as vitamin E, stress, and hormonal imbalances. (Of course, ***everything and anything is worse with stress***, amiright?!)

In conclusion, the liver is innocent! Let's stop calling them liver spots. Unless you have one that is really shaped like a liver. That might be kind of cute. Let's just keep it simple and call them sunspots. (But if you're dressed up for a fancy occasion, then I suppose whip out the "solar lentigines.")

29

DAY 29: THE SUGAR THING

WELL, it's day 29, and I've waited 'til the end to bring up the dreaded subject of **sugar and alcohol**.

By this point, I'm sure that you have already naturally reduced your intake of sugar and alcohol just by way of mindfulness and thinking about the liver bank!

Everybody knows about the downsides of alcohol. so we don't really need to get into that here.

But it still always seems like a bit of a buzz kill when someone starts talking about the evils of sugar.

It's not even that sugar is "bad."

Sugar is good!

You need it!

You just don't need so much of it.

Nature never meant for us to have such easy access to large amounts of sugar!

The sad truth is that excess sugar is probably the most common **dietary** contributor to liver trouble.

(The top cause of acute liver failure in the U.S. is actually acetaminophen - aka Tylenol - overdose, and alcohol abuse is definitely the most common cause of liver disease.)

If you're in a sugar addiction mode, then the thought of reducing your sugar intake is probably downright *painful!*

It feels like **life** will literally lose its sweetness!

But don't worry.

This is an illusion coming from the addiction.

Your taste buds are very adaptable, and they change over time as your diet changes.

Have you even been off the sugar before?

If you avoid it all together for a couple of weeks, then fruits start to taste almost like candy!

And if/when you do eat some candy, it's almost sickening.

If you can reduce your sugar intake, food will naturally begin to taste more flavorful.

The opposite is also true, and this is why we have to be careful when using artificial sweeteners.

Most artificial sweeteners are many times sweeter than sugar.

Even **stevia**, which is natural, is **200-400 times sweeter** than sugar!

Why does this matter?

It matters because it changes the sensitivity of the taste buds!

The taste buds become attuned to it, and then they end up craving much more "sweet" than before.

This is one way that people shoot themselves in the foot when they are trying to reduce their calories by choosing the "sugar free" options that are artificially sweetened.

(And now you're probably starting to see why "bitter" is such a good counterbalance to the stress that "sweet" can put onto the liver!)

It's a losing battle to say, "I just won't ever eat sugar again!"

Some people can pull it off, just like some people make it to the Olympics! But it's just not realistic for most of us average folks.

So, without judgement, just know that **healthy liver living means cutting down on the sugar intake!** And when you fall off the wagon, don't despair, judge or beat yourself up. Just look at that balance sheet and figure out how to make enough deposits to get back into the black!

It's a cliché, but it's true: **health is a journey, not a destination!**

Let me know how you're feeling about cutting back on sugar and/or alcohol!

Give your liver a pat and let it know that tomorrow is Graduation Day!

～

SHAMELESS SELF-PROMOTION
ABOUT THAT SUGAR THING...

SO, guess what? As I'm wrapping up this book, I've just finished the first round of my newest email course: The 21-Day Sugar Challenge!

Some of the Liver Challenge graduates specifically asked for a sugar-related program, so I made it happen! Feedback has been positive, and a lot of people have already asked for an extended version of the Sugar Challenge, and honestly, it makes sense! After all, sugar is a huge topic—there's no way to cover it thoroughly in just 21 days!

But I wanted to offer something "short" because a lot of people are intrigued by these challenges, but 30 days can sound like a long time. If you were one of those brave souls who jumped into the Liver Challenge with both feet, then this is right up your alley!

One of the greatest compliments so far may be this one that just came in this morning:

"This is such an introvert-friendly way to learn!"

. . .

And I have to say, I do fancy myself a Champion of Introverts everywhere!

Will there always be a book like this that goes along with every 30-Day Challenge program? Who knows? Time will tell!

Anyway, the sugar program can be found at

https://www.drkimsf.com/sugar

30

DAY 30: GRADUATION DAY

YOU DID IT!

Congratulations on making it to Day 30 of the challenge!

How did you do?

Take a moment to look back at your goals from the beginning. How do you feel compared to when you started?

How's your energy?
How's your thinking?
How's your mood?
How's your life?

Are you surprised at how much has changed just by focusing on taking care of your liver?

Most importantly... were you able to live your regular life without feeling like you were suffering or missing out compared to everyone else?

Today's challenge is simple: keep up with the great new habits you've developed.

Some strategies will work better for you than others, and that's okay.

You don't have to do everything—just focus on the best things.

Remember the 80/20 rule! The key is knowing which 20% of your efforts give you that 80% return!

And remember: nothing changes if nothing changes.

I know... sometimes, we wish we could make things change by magic.

Well, funny story... I happen to know a famous magician! He's often approached by people asking things like:

"How can I do magick to make the girl next door fall in love with me?"

And he always tells them:

"You can't.

You can only do magick on yourself, to become the kind of person the girl next door would fall in love with!"

And so it is with you on your journey toward health and happiness! You can't get new results by being the same person and doing the same things as before.

You have to become a new person, do new things... and then you get new results! That's how it works. There was nothing "wrong" with the old you. That was just a different person.

Kind of like how you think back to your 4th-grade self—That person was so different from who you are today! Nothing wrong with either one, they're just different. And now, you're going to be different again.

The only constant is change.

Do a little jump, pat your liver, and say, "Congrats! We did it!"

Thank you for taking this journey with me!

∼

Final Thoughts from the Author

These days, getting and staying healthy requires a lot of information! How can anyone remember it all?!

You can't.

That's why you need simple, constant reminders.

Lucky for you, I've got just the thing! It's called the **Daily Health Nugget**—a free daily email with a quick health tip or reminder.

No long reads, just a stick figure (because who has time to read *another* email, and honestly, I can't draw) with a short health tip underneath.

Subscribe to the Daily Health Nugget:

www.dailyhealthnugget.com

31

BONUS CHAPTER: THE (IN)FAMOUS LIVER FLUSH

WHEN I MENTIONED that I was putting together a 30-day Liver Challenge, someone asked me if I was going to include The Liver Flush.

Erm... No.

It's not that it doesn't work. It'll clean out those pipes all right! But... it's not my place to tell random strangers to do it. Unlike adequate hydration and a good night's sleep, it's not for everyone.

Years ago, I was having dinner with a colleague and his wife, and we were talking about The Liver Flush.

"Oh," he said, "I never recommend that to anyone anymore. No way."

"Why not?" I asked.

His wife then chimed in.

"Because I had to go to the hospital after I did it!"

Yikes! What happened?! She couldn't stop throwing up! She

ended up OK and did not need any intensive treatment, but still. It's not something you ever want to set someone up for!

So what is it, and why am I even bringing it up if I'm not going to tell you how to do it?!

Because there's a funny story to tell, and what better place to tell it than in the liver book?!

How did I even learn about it?

I learned about it in Hulda Clark's book, The Cure for All Diseases. I first encountered this book in the waiting area of Dr. Pesto's* office. (*not his real name) Dr. Pesto was my early mentor and arch nemesis. I worked as an independent contractor in his office for my first 2 years in San Francisco. There were 2 books that patients loved to look at while they were waiting. The big astrology book and The Cure for All Diseases.

That book actually has some good information in it. And that is also what makes it a potentially dangerous book. Because along with the good information, there is also a lot of dubious information.

Hulda Clark herself was a questionable character. She was a successful naturopath who – no doubt – helped a lot of people. She also likely scammed a lot of people. The many lawsuits and the arrest following a sting operation are clues. After examining the sting officer, she told them that they had HIV but that she could cure it! Then, after realizing it was a setup, she said that she'd made a mistake on the diagnosis. You can read about it online.

Anyway, Dr. Pesto encouraged me to read the book and to take the advice. I love to read, and I was game for anything, so I did.

I'm the kind of person who doesn't feel good telling other people to try something if I haven't tried it myself. So I tried many of the things recommended in that book!

One of the things that Dr. Clark touted was a device she called The Zapper. It's a little gadget that emits an electrical current at a specific frequency. It's basically a box with a battery and on/off switch and a couple of wires leading to 2 pieces of metal. You hold one of the metal pieces in each hand so that your body completes the circuit. (One of the lawsuits against Dr. Clark was from a man with a pacemaker. He went into dangerous arrhythmias after using The Zapper!) According to Dr. Clark, this is supposed to kill bacteria, viruses, and parasites.

Shortly after leaving Dr. Pesto's practice, I went to a seminar where they were selling some Zappers! They told me that no, the Zapper doesn't really work against viruses and bacteria. But it is excellent against parasites! And they claimed that theirs were the best. So, what the hell – I bought two. One for me, one for the office. I thought they were a bit pricey, but I had to know.

I couldn't feel any electrical current at all through the hand holds. I couldn't tell whether it was doing anything at all. Was it killing my parasites? What exactly were my parasites anyway?? I didn't know.

But I was fascinated by the idea, and I became a bit of a Zapper connoisseur. I started ordering other people's Zappers to compare. Were some of them effective? More economically priced? (I think that Hulda Clark even published a schematic for how to build your own Zapper.) Some of them did seem to be a little more intense than my first one. But I still couldn't tell if there was anything therapeutic happening in my body. I just went with it. I had a tiny "Micro Zapper" and one with huge hand holds that looked like sticks of dynamite.

Yeah, about that one with the dynamite-looking sticks...It was April 1, 2004.

The Iraq War was still new, but the War on Terror had been in full effect for years. My brother, a Marine, was still serving in Iraq. He had been on the ground when Saddam's palace was overtaken! He probably wasn't supposed to, but he picked up some souvenirs from the palace. Some stickers with an emblem of an eagle with swords jutting out and forming part of the wings. Some blank Ba'ath Party membership certificates. He gave me some of these.

My son was still a baby at the time. And my partner and I thought it would be hilarious if we put his picture on the certificate and hung it on the wall! (There is a little square on the certificate where the member's picture goes.)

If any of you have kids, you know what a ... rough time... that first year can be. Maybe it's different for extroverts, but for an awful lot of introverts, it sucks donkey balls. You don't sleep much, your house is a disaster zone, and you're doing good to shower on the regular! Some of the ladies out there might be able to relate to my main home outfit that year.

While I dutifully put on my classic skeleton t-shirt for work, home was a different story. I was usually rotating between two pieces of "sleepwear." I'm not even sure what they are officially called. Nursing gowns? One of them was a short (above the knee) cotton/poly blend thing with 2 easy-access boob flaps for nursing.

That's what I was wearing the morning of April 1, 2004. It was one day before my son's 1st birthday.

We were living at a condo complex with a security desk. People had to pass through security before they could come up and knock on the door. That morning, the security desk called and told me that two U.S. Marshalls were here to see me. I'm not sure what I thought I heard. Someone named Marshall?

"I don't know anyone named Marshall. Must be a wrong number. It's not me!" and I hung up.

The phone rang again.

It was the security desk again. U.S. Marshalls are here to see you.

"What do you mean? U.S. Marshalls like... THE Marshalls? For ME? Are you sure?"

"Is your name Kim?"

"Yes?"

"OK, well they're here to see you."

As I was waiting for them to make their way up to the apartment, I wracked my brain. What was this all about? There was no way that actual U.S. Marshalls could be coming up for ME! What the hell did I do?!

Buncha nothing, that's what!

I'd been basically disheveled and depressed with a baby for the last year! It was April 1, after all – maybe someone had sent me a gag singing telegram, meant to freak me out and then cheer me up! It had to be a singing telegram.

Finally, there was a knock on the door. I didn't have time to change. Plus I was bewildered. So I opened the door, standing there with troll pencil hair, barefoot and in my sad short nursing gown. And I looked at them. There was a short mean looking white guy and a tall mellow looking Black guy. The tall guy was wearing a black trench coat, and they both looked like they could be characters from Men in Black. Had to be a singing telegram! I waited for them to burst into song.

They did not burst into song.

"Can we come in?"

"Sure!" was my impulsive answer. (My partner later gave me hell for that. "YOU NEVER LET IN COPS!" he said. All I could think was, "What, are they like vampires?")

As they stepped into the hallway, my heart started to beat faster. I suddenly remembered the Ba'ath Party membership certificate on the wall. The one with my son's picture pasted onto it! Gah!!!!!

"Are you expecting something from Florida?" they asked.

"Uh... I dunno... like what?"

I searched my brain for what it could be. I might have been on a bit of an eBay binge around that time. I was ordering all sorts of crap. Mostly rocks and crystals, I think!

They asked again.

"Did you order something from Florida?"

"I order a lot of things... from eBay. Maybe something's coming from Florida? I don't know!"

The little mean white guy did most of the talking and zero of the smiling. I don't remember exactly what else they asked about. But in the end, the tall Black guy gave me his card and said, "You need to come down to the office. We have your package, and we have some questions."

Thankfully, they didn't say anything about the Ba'ath certificate on the wall. My son came crawling around the corner. I wonder if that's why they didn't make me come with them immediately to go down for questioning! I was so freaked out. I was too soft for prison! What would I do? What DID I do?!

I arranged for someone to come over and watch the baby while I went over to the U.S. Marshalls office to face my fate! It was just a 2-block walk from home. That's how they intercepted my package in the first place. Our mail was processed in the Federal Building's basement post office. This meant that every package was run through their x-ray machine!

When I got to the Marshalls floor, I was sent to a big conference room to wait. Then, an Asian agent came in with an opened Priority Mail box. The casting of the characters really did make it feel like I was in a movie. He laid out the contents on the table.

"You can see why we called you in." he said.

I breathed a sigh of relief and even laughed.

"For a Zapper??"

"What is it?" he asked.

I was embarrassed to say... because even then, I knew it was nutty...

"Umm... well, it's called a Zapper... it's supposed to kill parasites... but it probably doesn't! I know it's not FDA approved! I'm not using it on patients! Are they illegal??"

I was babbling like an idiot, and I knew with 100% certainty in that moment that I could have never made it as a spy. I would have crumbled under pressure and spilled every last bean. They wouldn't have even had to bring out the tray of surgical instruments and power tools to intimidate me! All they would have needed was one of those credit-card-sized multi-tools that goes in your wallet. They could point it menacingly at my fingernails and that would be enough!

I tried to explain how it "worked." And that I was kind of a collector of weird health gadgets. And how I was just looking for low prices on eBay. And how could I have known that it looked exactly like a pipe bomb?!

The guy heaved a heavy sigh and looked at me and said, "I mean... you can see why this was flagged, right? Two big pipes with wires that lead to a little box with a switch that just says ON?"

"Yes." I nodded, vowing to never order another eBay Zapper again!

He shrugged and stood up to leave.

"Can I keep my Zapper?" I asked.

"Sure," he said. "But please be mindful of what you order in the future."

I see that now, in 2022, they make Hulda Clark Zappers with a new modern design. Instead of the old timey hand holds, you can get tiny ones with metal plates that you touch with your fingertips. I won't be trying them out, though. The whole Federal Marshalls at the door thing was a bit of a buzz kill. Plus, I think they might be bullshit.

Anyway, I can't remember whether "zapping" was supposed to come before or after the legendary Liver Flush, but that was the whole initial intent. I had been plagued with vague "liver stress" for years. Dr. Pesto strongly recommended that I do some liver flushing.

And since I don't recommend things that I haven't tried myself, I tried them all. I did gentle "liver flushes" that involved daily shots of raw garlic mixed with lemon juice and olive oil. I've done the one that uses copious amounts of whipped cream in place of the olive oil. I've done the classic Epsom salt and olive oil one many times. And I even attempted a "simple" version that just used supplements but ended up causing projectile vomiting! That was my very first experience with projectile vomiting. (My assistant at the time also attempted that "supplement flush" and also experienced the same projectile vomiting! Not sure if either of us "flushed" anything from our livers, but... we shredded that recipe, never to speak of it again!)

The whole point of "liver flushing" is to clear out the bile ducts, which can get clogged with thick greasy deposits. If you've done it successfully, you will see the evidence in the toilet! It usually looks like tons of tiny green pebbles, mostly smaller than a pea. Once, an old lady brought me some frozen poop in a Tupperware container to ask whether the little green things in there were the "liver stones." Yep, that was them. (I know they are not actual "stones" – that is just what they are called.)

I've seen a lot of people experience immediate benefits following a successful flush. The most common things are better mood, less pain, better digestion, and headache relief.

I believe that some of my liver flushing from back then helped to prevent gallstones later in life. The reason for this is that one day, after my 3rd liver flush, I noticed a strange looking "stone."

It looked different from the other ones. It was a little bigger and more pale in color. Being the scientifically inclined person that I am, I grabbed a glove and poked it. It was not greasy like the green ones. It had a hard shell! I pressed harder, and the shell cracked! It freaked me out! That thing seemed to be calcifying! Whatever it was, it really was turning into a stone! Yikes! I was glad to have it out of my body before it got any bigger.

Liver flushes are a funny thing. Once you do it, you suddenly want to talk to other people who've done it, too, so that you can compare notes! It's a really strange club.

Anyway, I could go on with liver flush stories. But since they are essentially poop stories, I think I should just save it... for the poop book.

∾

ABOUT BOOKS THAT SAVE LIVES

Books That Save Lives came into being in 2024 when the editor and publisher, Brenda Knight, heard directly from readers and authors that certain self-help, grief, psychology books, and journals were providing a lifeline for folks. We live in a stressful world where it is increasingly difficult not to feel overwhelmed, worried, depressed, and downright scared. We intend to offer support for the vulnerable, including people struggling with mental wellness and physical illness as well as people of color, queer and trans adults and teens, immigrants and anyone who needs encouragement and inspiration.

From first responders, military veterans, and retirees to LGBTQ+ teens and to those experiencing the shock of bereavement and loss, our books have saved lives. To us, there is no higher calling.

We would love to hear from you! Our readers are our most important resource; we value your input, suggestions, and ideas.
Please stay in touch with us and follow us at:
www.booksthatsavelives.net
https://www.instagram.com/booksthatsavelives/